Fingergym™

Fine Motor Skills

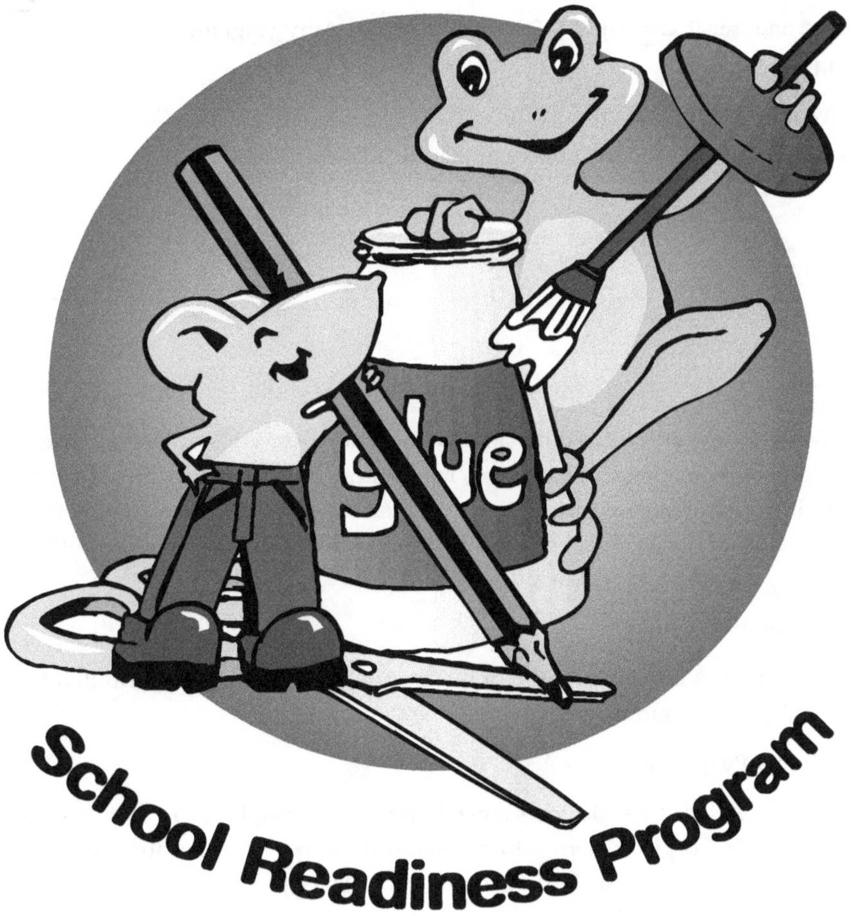

School Readiness Program

Gayle Brook | Amy Wagenfeld | Cathy Thompson

First published in 2006 by
Australian Academic Press
32 Jeays Street
Bowen Hills QLD 4006
Australia
www.australianacademicpress.com.au

ISBN-13: 9781875378753

Illustrations by Jill Lincoln.

Music composed by Toby Thompson.

Cover and text design by Andrea Rinarelli of Australian Academic Press.

For Jessica and Sarah and
in memory of my Dad, James Edbrooke
Gayle

For David
Amy

For all the children who have been part of Fingergym™
over the years, with a special mention to the children
of Patricks Road State Primary School, Queensland, Australia
Cathy

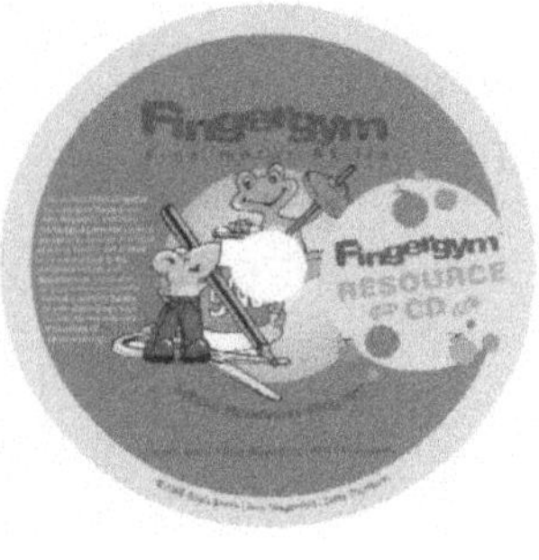

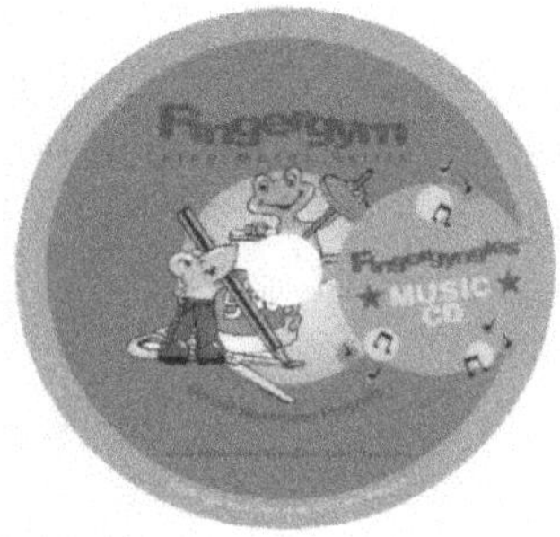

Where are my CDs?

Fingergym was first released in 2006 when CDs were often used to include extra program resources with printed books. Times have changed. Today, many computers exclude CD/DVD players. Therefore we have taken the decision to move the contents of both the Fingergym Resources CD and Fingergym Music CD to secure online digital storage.

Using either the url or QR code links below, the purchaser is permitted to download and save the data and music files on a secure digital storage platform. A permanent licence is granted to the purchaser to print out all the data and play the music files in part or whole on an unlimited basis for the purchaser's own non-profit educational use.

The contents of all downloads remains the copyright of Gayle Brook, Amy Wagenfeld, and Cathy Thompson.

Fingergym Data CD contents

https://sowl.co/bwBF2y

Fingergym Music CD contents

https://sowl.co/zEYut

Contents

About the Authors

Gayle Brook, BoccThy, ATCL (Speech & Drama), is a private practitioner in Brisbane, Australia with a special interest in helping children discover their own learning potential. A graduate of The University of Queensland, Australia in 1988, she gained experience as a student in Toronto, Canada and also worked in South Carolina, United States. She has worked in schools and in private practice since returning to Australia in 1991. Gayle enjoys incorporating drama and lots of fun fine motor activities into her occupational therapy sessions. Gayle is married and the mother of two beautiful girls.

Amy Wagenfeld, PhD, OTR/L, has practised occupational therapy for over 20 years, working in such areas as gerontology and rehabilitation, and for the past 15 plus years in paediatrics. She has earned a BS in occupational therapy, an MA in human development, and a PhD in early childhood education. Amy currently teaches at a Boston area college in the United States of America, provides school-based consultative services, and maintains a private practice. Amy lives in suburban Boston with her husband and terrific son.

Cathy Thompson enjoys helping children with special needs and has worked in education for over 12 years. Currently employed as a research assistant at Queensland University of Technology, her career background includes devising and running intervention programs for children with physical impairments and learning difficulties, and running gymnastics programs for local authorities in the United Kingdom and Australia.

Acknowledgments

This program has been a work in progress for many years. Thanks must go to our families for being understanding about time spent away from them while plugging away at our computers. Also, thanks to those who have encouraged us to pursue our dream of writing and publishing this program, even when the 'going got tough'.
Amy and Gayle

I would like to acknowledge the support and encouragement of the following people: my husband David; my children Sam, Toby, and Emily; Cecilia Webb, Lyndal O'Gorman, Barbara McKinlay, and Gayle Brook.
Cathy

Thanks to Toby Thompson for his musical contribution to the *Fingergyngles*™ CD and technical 'wizardry'.

Thanks also to the talented editorial staff at Australian Academic Press.

Finally, thanks must go to all of the children and teachers who have been part of trialling the activities in the Fingergym™ program.

Preface

We are delighted that you have chosen to add the *Fingergym™ Fine Motor Skills School Readiness Program* to your classroom library. We hope that you find it to be an easy-to-use and helpful resource for you and your students.

We would like to share with you how the program originated and developed. We (Amy and Gayle) met 16 years ago when we were both temporarily living and working as occupational therapists in Columbia, South Carolina, and we have maintained an ongoing written friendship and collegial relationship ever since. Gayle now lives in Brisbane, Australia and Amy resides in Boston, United States of America.

What began as Gayle's project to compile a simple book of fine motor activities for teachers at her daughter's school became a collaborative and connected work, completed almost entirely through electronic communication.

At a later stage in the development of the program Cathy Thompson, an innovative teacher aide, came on board to provide valuable insight and hands-on experience as to how these activities could be incorporated into a small group program, which she had developed and called Fingergym™.

It is our hope that through books and programs such as this the world of occupational therapy, education, and child development will also become closer and more linked as we work towards the common goal of educating our young children.

Gayle Brook
Amy Wagenfeld
Cathy Thompson

An Introduction to the Fingergym™ Program

'Fingergym™ is all about trying'
(Jack, age 5)

A hesitant little boy walked slowly into the room, wondering what was going to be expected of him now. For much of the morning he had sat at his desk, trying to remember how to hold his scissors and cut on the big black lines, listen to the teacher, and remember where to glue the picture and make his fingers hold the pencil to write his name at the top of the page. All of these tasks required multiple skills that this little boy hadn't yet mastered, and he felt sad and wished that he could do these things easily like his friends.

Then he heard the music and a familiar voice saying, 'Hi kids! Welcome to Fingergym ...', and he knew that for just a little while he could practise all those 'tricky' things in a safe and encouraging place, where he could experience success and feel free to just have a go.

The *Fingergym™ Fine Motor Skills School Readiness Program* is a unique, classroom-trialled, small group rotation program that uses fun and motivating fine motor–based activities and a self-directing music CD called *Fingergyngles™* (Now available as a digital download — see page iv) to target many of the wide array of skills necessary to help children become more independent in the classroom environment. It was developed by two occupational therapists working in two different countries and a teacher aide with 12 years' experience that includes devising and planning intervention programs for children with physical impairments.

In addition to focusing on fine motor skills, the program also promotes the development of **school readiness skills**, such as the ability to:

- organise work space and tools
- maintain a sitting position
- be aware of other people and their needs
- follow visual and auditory directions
- ask for help if needed
- initiate and complete a task
- problem-solve and actively investigate cause and effect situations
- transition from one task to another

- maintain attention
- risk take or have a go.

These readiness skills, which are by no means all inclusive, are important because as educators we know that being ready for school and coping in the classroom involves so much more on the part of the child than just being able to hold a pencil, cut along a line, or glue a picture.

The Fingergym™ program promotes development of fine motor and school readiness skills by providing the child with regular opportunities to practise in a safe and supportive environment. Because the program is consistently set up the same way, children know what to expect and become more confident to have a go. The rotational nature of the program and the consistent 'timed' frequency of the activities encourages children to listen carefully for the instructions, work out a 'plan' to do the task or ask for help quickly if they do not know what to do, and stay focused in order to complete the task. Although the fine motor activities are supportive of other classroom fine motor tasks, the underlying philosophy of the program is that children are encouraged to problem-solve, have a go, and keep trying without the added pressure of producing an academic product.

By incorporating play-based learning this program focuses on the process of learning through exploration, with the aim of enhancing developmental skills, including fine motor and school readiness skills. For example, a child doing a treasure hunt activity with chopsticks is unaware that she is doing a task to help develop a mature tripod pencil grasp. In her mind she is just having fun being involved in a play-based exploration activity. However, in addition to working on the skills needed to be ready to hold her pencil correctly, along the way in her Fingergym™ program she has also practised the following skills:

- Listening — she has listened to the teacher give the instructions.
- Initiation and self-control — she waited for the Fingergyngles™ music to begin while seating herself at the activity station.
- Focusing and, as much as possible, independently completing a task — she performed the task until the music began again.
- Remembering and self-monitoring — she remembered how to hold her chopsticks and adjusted her fingers to do it like the teacher showed her.
- Organising workspace — she quickly packed away the chopsticks.
- Being aware of the needs of others — she waited patiently for Johnny, who was a little slower than herself in moving to the next station.

The Fingergym™ program promotes an organised and dynamic five-point learning system, which requires each child to:

- **Think:** Develop a plan ('How do I do this activity?')
- **Initiate:** Start the activity
- **Focus:** Stay on the activity
- **Finish:** Complete the activity
- **Transition:** Move to the next activity.

The program has been successfully implemented with:

- children who have already been assessed by an occupational therapist and are participating in a fine motor program outside of the classroom or school
- children in kindergarten and preschool and prep-aged children identified by teachers as demonstrating difficulty with fine motor skills, including reluctance to use a pencil or ineffective use of other school tools
- children with specific diagnosed disorders, including intellectual impairment, speech and language impairment, autistic spectrum disorder, and attention-deficit/hyperactivity disorder

- children with fine motor weakness due to limited experience or opportunities to practise at home
- children with mild sensory integration problems, such as poor crossing of the midline of the body or tactile defensiveness
- children with visual convergence and eye-tracking problems
- children displaying anxiety over attempting new or challenging activities
- children displaying difficulty organising themselves, their belongings, or equipment
- children displaying difficulty in starting a task, staying on a task, or transitioning smoothly from one task to another
- children who have difficulty following instructions
- children displaying postural weakness or generally lacking in strength and endurance
- children demonstrating self-care difficulties with buttons, zips, shoelaces, and other fasteners.

For further information and updates on the Fingergym™ program go to www.fingergym.info

Ten-Step Countdown to Fingergym™

This checklist was specially developed for teachers and teacher aides who are responsible for getting the Fingergym™ program started in their school or centre. Read carefully through each step and tick it off when the task has been completed. It is recommended that you follow each step, as this will ensure you set up for the program with minimum fuss and maximum efficiency.

☐ **Step 1**. (IMPORTANT) Read Fine Motor Development and Early School Performance to gain an overview of fine motor skill development and the underlying philosophy and principles of this program. *Ensure that helpers also read this section.

☐ **Step 2**. Read Running the Fingergym™ Program thoroughly to ensure that you are familiar with the different program formats, which will assist you in choosing the best program for your student and classroom needs and resources.

☐ **Step 3**. Based on your classroom and student needs, choose your program format:

____

☐ **Step 4**. Familiarise yourself with the activities in Section B.

Hint: The activity checklists on the resource CD might be helpful for you to keep note of activities for which you already have the necessary resources, or those that would be most appropriate to implement with your students. These checklists will be especially useful if you are preparing your own activity schedule.

☐ **Step 5**. Follow the sample activity schedule on the resource CD.

OR

Use the blank schedule on the resource CD to develop your own activity schedule.

☐ **Step 6**. Photocopy, cut out, and laminate the activity cards you have chosen for your program.

☐ **Step 7**. Place the activity cards, together with the activity equipment, into zipper-top storage bags and store in a box with activities from the same category, such as strengthening. Alternatively, you can store your activity cards in a small filing box under the differently labelled headings.

☐ **Step 8**. Print out and photocopy relevant forms or templates on the resource CD, for example, parent information/permission letters, Trainers Mud Map, and activity templates.

☐ **Step 9**. For easy access, file the forms into a three-ring binder complete with visibly labelled clear plastic inserts.

☐ **Step 10**. Get ready to start your program!

Section A
Fingergym™ Overview

This section contains supporting theory about fine motor development and early school performance, and detailed information about how to set up for and run the program.

Fine Motor Development and Early School Performance

WHAT ARE FINE MOTOR SKILLS?

Fine motor skills are the collective skills and activities that involve using the hands and fingers (Amundson & Weil, 2001; Case-Smith & Shortridge, 1996). That is, fine motor skills are those skills that require the small muscles of the hand to work together to perform precise and refined movements.

WHEN DO FINE MOTOR SKILLS DEVELOP?

Fine motor skills typically develop in a reasonably consistent and predictable pattern in the early years of childhood (from birth through to mid primary school; Exner, 2001). The process begins in infancy when a 2- to 3-month-old baby first bats at a toy, then progresses to grasping, releasing, and transferring objects between their hands (Case-Smith & Shortridge, 1996; Edwards, Buckland, & McCoy-Powlen, 2002; Erhardt, 1994). They then progress to using fingers to manipulate and explore things, stack blocks, self-feed, and dress, and during the early childhood years use 'school tools' such as scissors, markers, crayons, pencils, and glue.

By the time a child enters Grade 1, there are a number of fine motor skills that they generally demonstrate in a spontaneous and well-integrated manner. Depending on the child's previous experience and exposure to different activities, the quality of these skills varies. However, with age, ongoing experience, and practice, the quality of each child's fine motor skills continues to develop throughout childhood.

However, none of these fine motor skills can develop smoothly without the concurrent development of gross motor (large muscle) skills. In fact, typically, development proceeds in a cephalo–caudal (head to toe) and proximal–distal (moving from the body parts closest to the trunk to those furthest away) pattern (Gesell & Amatruda, 1947). That is why it is important to include things like 'tummy time' for infants, to encourage development of their trunk, shoulder, and hip musculature. In simple terms, this means that development of stable shoulders and upper arms provides a solid base for the development of skills such as self-feeding and using scissors and writing tools. Likewise, without well-developed hip and trunk musculature, sitting upright in a chair becomes quite challenging.

Early developmental skills and milestones work together to provide a solid foundation for the more integrated motor skills required in upper grades. These higher-level skills include being able to write fluently and focus on writing content (such as conveying information, thoughts, and ideas) rather than on the mechanics of writing, which involves pencil grasp, letter formation, spacing, and sizing. Figure 1 shows the progression of typical fine motor development.

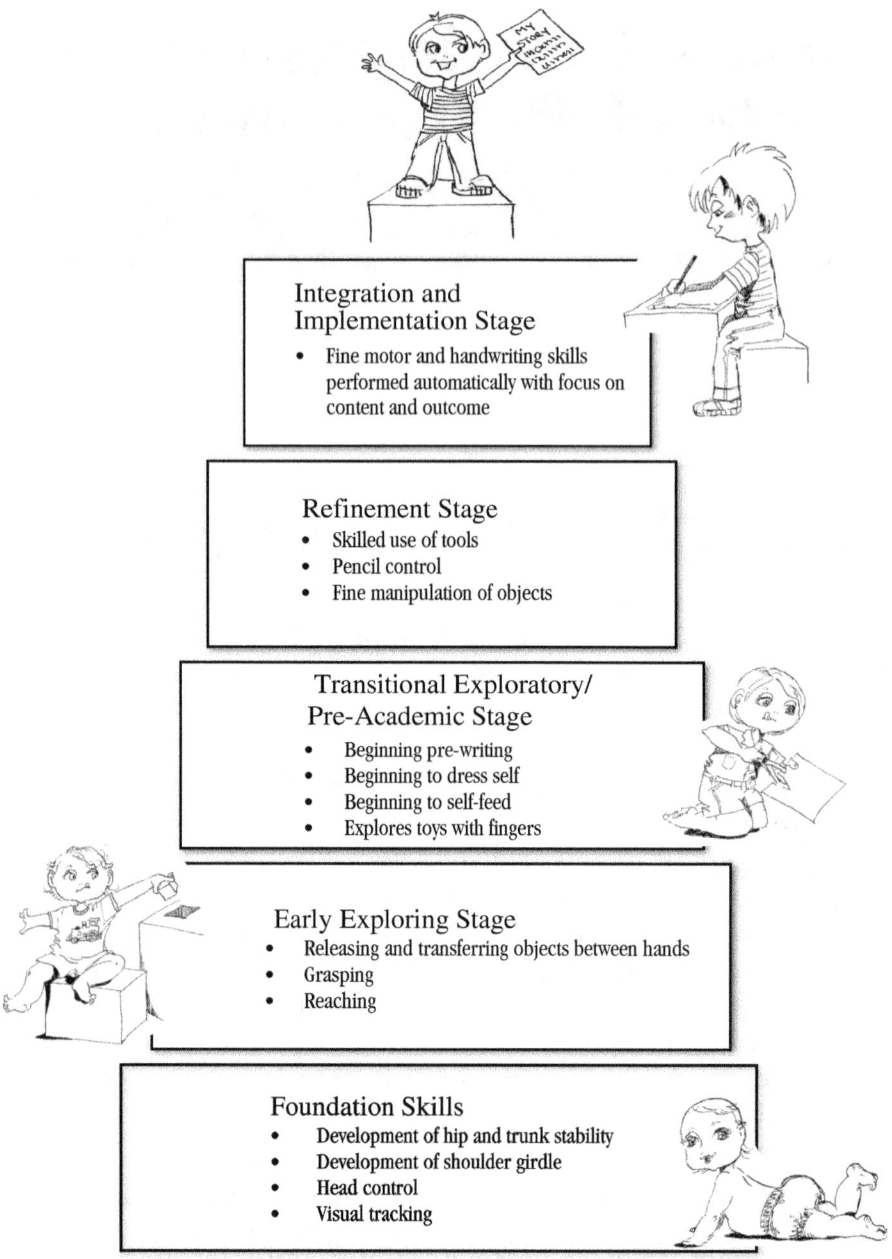

Figure 1. A Bottom–Up Hierarchy and Progression of Typical Fine Motor Development

WHAT FINE MOTOR SKILLS SHOULD CHILDREN BE DEVELOPING TO GET READY FOR FORMAL SCHOOLING?

In the preschool years, the foundational skills developed in infancy and toddler-hood are being built upon as a child *readies* to use school tools. Although many kindergarten-aged children are fascinated with scissors, crayons, markers, and such, writing and cutting should not be the main focus of fine motor work for 3- to 4-year-olds. It is often more beneficial to use this time of readiness to create a foundation for future school tool use (Yakimishyn & Magill-Evans, 2002). In fact, at this age some children may be extremely reluctant to even pick up a pencil. For these children, it is far better to encourage them to participate in related activities that support the development of the hand and finger muscles needed to correctly hold and use pencils and scissors rather than force them to do writing activities before they are ready. Such related activities might include:

- picking up objects using oversized tongs and tweezers
- activating and playing with wind-up toys
- spinning small hand-held tops

- popping bubble plastic with thumb and index finger
- drawing in the sand with a stick, feather, or straw
- using clothes pegs to help hang up clothes or pictures
- using squirt guns or squeeze-trigger containers (a great way to get windows clean!).

WHAT FINE MOTOR SKILLS CAN BE EXPECTED FROM A CHILD ENTERING SCHOOL?

Children in the first year of school present with varying skill levels, ranging from having highly developed fine motor skills, such as proficient pencil skills, to having very definite 'gaps' in their fine motor skills, such as being unable to use scissors or having an inefficient or immature pencil grasp. However, the fine motor skills that *typically developing* 5- to 6-year-olds progressing from preschool or prep to school generally demonstrate are quite amazing and include the ability to:

- demonstrate hand dominance
- use the tips of the fingers and the thumb together in a precise pinch or pincer grasp
- assume and use some form of tripod pencil grasp, where a writing tool is held between the tips of the thumb, index finger, and middle finger (versus a whole hand grasp)
- follow an object smoothly with the eyes only while the head remains still
- cut around reasonably complex designs such as a combination of straight and curved lines and corners, with less than 0.5 cm deviation from set lines
- draw a circle, triangle, square, and recognisable picture of a person and a house
- use one hand to stabilise an object and the other to perform a separate activity such as unscrewing a lid and doing up buttons, and think of the stabilising hand as the *helper* hand and the hand performing the task as the *worker* hand
- manipulate small objects within the hand
- put together a complex, interlocking puzzle
- independently complete many self-care tasks such as simple dressing, toileting, shoelace tying, and lunch set-up (Beery, 1997; Brigance, 1978; Case-Smith & Shortridge, 1996; Edwards, Buckland, & McCoy-Powlen, 2002; Exner, 1989; Exner, 2001; Furuno et al., 1987; Shaffer, 2002).

WHAT IMPACT MIGHT WEAK FINE MOTOR SKILLS HAVE ON A CHILD?

For some children, their hands do not seem to work together in the way that they should (Woodward & Swinth, 2002). This may lead to such frustration that they may resist activities that require them to coordinate all of the muscles and joints in their hands and fingers. As a result, they do not get to practise these skills correctly or develop the correct muscles (Woodward & Swinth, 2002). This in turn may affect the development of higher-level fine motor skills, such as writing. It is often at the stage when formal handwriting instruction has commenced that children are identified as having fine motor weakness (Amundson & Weil, 2001; Dennis & Swinth, 2001). Resultant commonly seen behaviours might include:

- outright refusal to participate in an activity
- avoidance techniques ('I need to get a drink of water')
- anger outbursts (rip up paper / tantrums)
- sadness (crying)
- 'defeatist' behaviour ('I'm no good, I can't do this').

Further, research suggests that children and adolescents with identified motor coordination weakness are at higher risk of experiencing anxiety and even depression associated with their perceived lack of competence in motor activities (Losse et al., 1991; Skinner & Piek, 2001). Therefore, it is important for teachers and parents to be aware of the impact that fine motor skill performance, or a child's perception of their own fine motor performance in relation to their peers', may have on the child's overall behaviour in the classroom. Working to help children develop the best fine motor skills possible at a young age helps to set the stage for success in school and at home, and also contributes to them feeling good about themselves. It also has huge run-off benefits for teachers who can then concentrate on teaching concepts of information rather than focusing on the mechanics of cutting, gluing, or writing.

WHAT CAN TEACHERS DO TO HELP?

It is important for teachers to identify those children who are most likely at risk of fine motor weakness as early as possible and to subsequently incorporate specific fine motor activities into those children's day. In fact, many children show significant improvement in their fine motor skills when given greater exposure to, and practice in, novel fine motor activities (Dankert, Davies, & Gavin, 2003; Marr, Cermak, Cohn, & Henderson, 2003).

Teachers may also play an important part in keeping children motivated to practise skills that they might find challenging. Maintaining a positive and upbeat demeanour and encouraging children to have a go may reduce the likelihood that they will view themselves as a failure and refuse to attempt fine motor tasks in the future. It may also be necessary to modify classroom tasks or reduce expectations until the children experiencing fine motor challenges have developed a greater sense of self-confidence and demonstrated an improved skills level.

However, it is important to remember that for some children fine motor dysfunction may only be part of a broader developmental delay. It is strongly recommended that those children who are identified as at risk be referred for more detailed assessment by an occupational therapist. In fact, when there is any question in your mind about whether a child's fine motor difficulties are part of a more global issue, consult with an occupational therapist. Remember, this book is not a substitute for occupational therapy services.

FREQUENTLY ASKED QUESTIONS

When is the best time to focus on fine motor skills?

If possible, carry out fine motor activities after a period of gross motor activities, those activities involving movement of the large muscle groups of the body such as the shoulders, upper arms, hips, and thighs (American Occupational Therapy Association, 1989), especially those requiring some weight bearing through the upper limbs. Fine motor activities initiated after a physical education session, or after a recess period when the children have been running around outside, works very well. This helps to 'awaken' the larger muscle groups and ready them to act as the support and stabilisers necessary for engagement in fine motor activities. Remember, warm-ups work. Creative movement and music are wonderful ways to warm up and prepare children to attend to fine motor work. Fine motor time is a natural lead-in for something academic.

Helpful hint

- If it is not possible to schedule fine motor activities following a period of gross motor play, try incorporating some strengthening activities within the classroom context, such as crab walks or push-ups from a sitting position or off a wall.

Should I make a big deal about how the children sit?

Children are sometimes referred for occupational therapy because of poor sitting posture. On observing these children in class, it is often discovered that they sit incorrectly due to a poor seating arrangement or incorrect desk or chair height and depth. Although it may turn out that there are other factors involved in poor posture, such as lowered muscle tone or sensory issues, look at these things first. Then, be sure the child's sitting posture is correct. This involves a number of factors, including:

- Feet should be flat on the floor. Use contact paper–covered old phone books or some other type of footrest if chair or desk height cannot be changed. Incorrect feet placement is one of the most common reasons for poor sitting posture at a desk.
- Hips should be back in the chair. Sometimes non-slip matting may help prevent the hips from sliding forward. Look at the depth of the seat. If children cannot sit comfortably with their hips positioned near the back of the chair, consider changing chairs or using a back bolster.
- Back should be reasonably straight in the chair.
- Hips, knees, and ankles should be at 90-degree angles to the floor.
- Face should be approximately at a forearm's distance from the work page or desk. To check for proper sitting position, remind children to place their elbows on the table and then place their face in their palm.
- Desktop should be approximately at elbow height.
- For the child experiencing extreme difficulty sitting in a standard desk chair, consider one with arms. This offers greater stability and provides sensory cues for body space awareness.
- Begin each session with the popular rhyme about sitting:
    - *1, 2, 3, 4 Are your feet flat on the floor?*
    - *5, 6, 7, 8 Is your back up tall and straight?*
    - *9, 10, 11, 12 Show me how your pencil is held.*

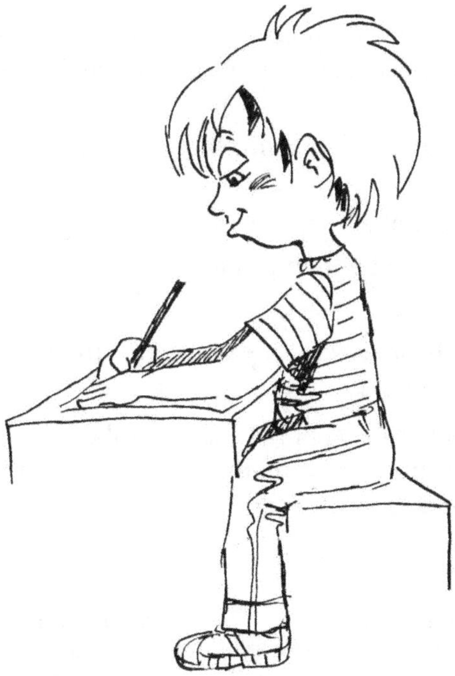

Helpful hints

Many children with lowered muscle tone in their hands will also have low muscle tone and strength throughout their body, including their trunk muscles. These are often the children that rest their heads in their hands, slump to one side, and just find it difficult to sit upright in their chairs.

- Try raising the desk height so that body and arms are more supported.
- Allow these children more frequent movement-oriented break times, and play wake-up games like Simon Says.
- Try placing an air-filled cushion such as a slightly inflated beach ball or commercially available gel- or air-filled cushion on the chair. This allows children some wiggling movement that does not disrupt others.

How do I cater to all the different levels of ability in a class?

Children with similar fine motor challenges or strengths may be grouped together, or a combination of children with different skill levels can be grouped together. Creating mixed skill–level groups or leading whole class activities involves more planning. However, by using grading techniques (see the How Can I Make the Activities in This Program Easier or Harder section below) it is possible to keep all children in the group focused.

Helpful hint

- For students with a short attention span or compliance difficulties, the music break on the *Fingergyngles*™ CD helps them realise that they do the task just for that set amount of time.

How can I make the activities in this program easier or harder?

Making an activity easier or harder is called grading (Shepherd, 2001). For many of the activities in this manual, suggestions for making the task harder (△) or easier (▽) have been included.

In general, the level of skill required for the activities can be *increased* in the following ways:

- introducing different tools, such as tweezers, kitchen tongs, ice-cube tongs, chopsticks, toothpicks, spoons, magnetic fishing rods, or different-sized crayons, pencils, or brushes
- increasing the amount of resistance in the task, for example, using clay instead of Play-Doh®, or introducing dough or clay containing mix-ins such as kosher salt crystals or coarse sand
- increasing the demand for accuracy, for example, drawing through a wide then increasingly narrow pathway
- increasing the speed and timing of an activity
- decreasing the size of the object to be manipulated
- increasing the number of repetitions
- increasing the complexity of the activity, for example, completing simple straight-line mazes followed by curved and angled ones.

To make a task *easier*, do the opposite to what is suggested above. For example, use tools that require a gross grasp rather than finer movements, or use large crayons or markers before introducing narrow pencils or markers.

Helpful hint

- Most regular activities can be made to be more exciting and motivating simply by using some of the above methods. Think liberally and laterally about activities that you are using, and then experiment. The children will love it.

What is more important, process or outcome?

Sometimes children may not seem to have any apparent fine motor difficulties when really they *are* having fine motor difficulties. For example, for some children, their colouring is neat and their cutting is accurate, but they still seem to strongly dislike doing fine motor tasks. A more in-depth, systematic look may reveal that they are having difficulties with the *process*, not the actual *outcome*, of fine motor work (Amundson & Weil, 2001). These children may be very slow to complete tasks, may be perfectionists, and may demonstrate hand fatigue through complaints of sore hands or frequent hand wringing or wriggling. As the skill-level requirements and speed for completing tasks increases with each grade, these children may become increasingly reluctant to write or use school tools such as glue, scissors, or a ruler. Therefore, it is important to do the following:

- Encourage these children to participate in fine motor activities and reassure them that it is okay if their work is not perfect. Praise *all* efforts.
- Change the fine motor focus in different sessions. For example, for children who cut slowly and 'over perfectly', one day have best cutting as a target and another day choose fast cutting as a target.
- Look at the quality and process of the fine motor skill, and not just the outcome, as the skill may not yet be functional and integrated. For example, a child may produce an accurately cut-out picture, but may have taken an excessive amount of time to complete it. Or, a child may accurately copy a letter but may not be able to reproduce that letter from visual memory.
- Identify the child's particular area of weakness or strength. In general, it may be easier to do this once a fine motor activity is broken down into its various tasks and components.

Running the Fingergym™ Program

PROGRAM MATERIALS

Manual

Included in this manual is supportive basic theory about the development of fine motor skills and how important the acquisition of these skills are to a child's early feelings of success in the classroom and overall early academic performance, different options for implementing the program in your own unique classroom situation, instructions on how to prepare and set up for the program, over 140 fine motor activities, and appendices containing the contents of the resource CD (all the support materials for the program), including thumbnail images of each file to assist with easy identification, and information about the field trials conducted on the program.

Fingergyngles™ CD

The *Fingergyngles™* CD accompanies the activities and assists the children to transition independently from one activity to the next with a catchy musical cue and the voices of two animal characters: Fidget the Frog™ and Mani the Mouse™. There are three tracks on the CD. Track 1 is an introductory track, and tracks 2 and 3 have different running times for the program: 16 minutes on Track 2 and 26 minutes on Track 3.

Resource CD

The resource CD contains all of the support materials for the program, such as templates for activities, awards, and information letters for parents. It is a valuable and time-saving resource for busy teachers; and the materials on it can be printed out as many times as you wish. The contents of the resource CD are also listed in the Appendix A of this manual, to assist with easy location of the files you are looking for.

DIFFERENT FORMATS FOR RUNNING THE PROGRAM

The program has been developed so that you can vary the format in which you run it, depending on your unique classroom situation. These options are outlined below. However, feel free to be creative with these options. For example, if you have a large number of children who will be participating in the program, you may choose to run the program in either of the small group formats with multiple small groups (that is, one small group completes the program and then another small group completes the program after the first, and so on) rather than run it in the whole class format.

Individual child

As it is optimal to begin with large muscle strengthening activities and work towards more refined ones, when running the program with an individual child the child begins at the strengthening station, completes the activity, and then moves to the next station at the musical cue. You may choose to remove the child from the classroom and set up the program in a distraction-free place, or place the child in a one-to-one situation with a trained program trainer within the classroom setting. The benefit of running the program with an individual child is that the child receives individual instruction and increased focus on his/her unique needs and goals.

Small group (individual rotation)

The small group with individual rotation format accommodates up to five children. Each child begins at a different activity station, completes the activity, and moves to the next station at the musical cue. It is best if this small group moves from the main classroom to a quiet, separate room or area. The benefits of running the program in this way are twofold. Single desks can be used so that each child can concentrate without distraction from other children working at the same table, and although each child individually participates at each station they are still part of a group dynamic. The small group with individual rotation option can be used to target at-risk children or children with an identified delay in fine motor development.

Small group rotation

The small group rotation format accommodates up to five children. All children and the trainer start together at the strengthening station, complete the activity, and at the musical cue move to the next station. This format requires a larger area, multiple pieces of equipment at each station, large tables that can accommodate five children, and more set-up. The benefits of running the program in this way are that it allows the trainer to move with the whole group to the next station, and allows the optimal principle of starting with large muscle strengthening activities and moving to more refined activities, such as cutting and pencil to paper tasks. This option may be used with specific children identified as experiencing fine motor and school readiness delays, or with a combination of children who are experiencing challenges and a few who are not. When organised thoughtfully, children who are not experiencing fine motor difficulties may serve as positive role models for those who need some special attention.

Whole class (small group rotation)

When running the program with the whole class with small group rotation, each small group goes to a different activity station. (Ensure that there is enough space for children to stand or sit around the tables.) The children complete the activity, and then, at the musical cue, move to the next station. For this format, enough materials are required at each activity station so that all of the children in each small group can perform the activity simultaneously, and so that all of the children in the class can perform the activity when it is their turn. For this approach, it is important that the program trainer is highly organised and has easy access to materials. A program trainer at each station would make this approach work smoothly. The benefits of running the program in this format are that the whole class can participate, and the teacher can be involved.

THINGS TO CONSIDER WHEN PLANNING TO RUN THE PROGRAM

Which children will be involved in the program?

Perhaps there are just a few children who seem to be struggling more than others with fine motor skills, or maybe the entire class does not manage fine motor tasks very confidently. By the end of the first term of the school year, most teachers will probably have a reasonable idea about which children are struggling with fine motor tasks. However, it is important to seriously consider the question of which children will be involved in the program before beginning the program.

Have the children in the class with specific fine motor and readiness skills weakness been identified?

If children with specific fine motor and readiness skills weakness have not already been identified, use the checklists provided on the resource CD to gain a basic profile of each child's fine motor strengths and weaknesses and readiness skills.

> **IMPORTANT**. These checklists will not give a comprehensive assessment of fine motor or readiness skills. If you have specific concerns about a child's fine motor or readiness skills, referral to an occupational therapist is advised. The occupational therapist will be able to identify specific areas of delay as well as underlying reasons for poor fine motor skills. For example, diminished muscle tone or strength in the hands may negatively affect pencil grasp. A specific program to help children improve areas of weakness while also taking into account identified areas of strength may then be designed and implemented in consultation with the occupational therapist, teachers, and parents. If there are other developmental concerns, such as language, attention, vision, or cognition, the relevant health professionals should also be consulted.

If the children who have specific fine motor and readiness skills weakness have been identified, consider what support they are receiving. Have they been formally assessed by an occupational therapist, or do you need to refer them to one? Also, consider whether it may be in order to suggest that the child receive a complete eye examination, as visual acuity and perceptual problems may negatively influence a child's fine motor skills.

Helpful hints

- Identify children with fine motor and readiness skills weakness.
- Refer appropriate children to an occupational therapist for detailed assessment.
- Refer children to other appropriate health professionals where indicated.
- Send a permission or information letter home to parents regarding their child's participation in the Fingergym™ program (see resource CD).

Which format should the program be run in?

After determining the number of children who will be participating and their level of need and supervision, choose the most appropriate format. It is suggested that children with more significant needs participate in the individual or small group (individual rotation) formats.

Helpful hint

- Choose the most suitable type of program format for your needs.

How often will the program be run?

Decide how frequently you can run the program. Remember, little and often works the best. Of course, daily application would be optimal; however, based on the results of teacher trials, *two to three* times a week is suggested as realistic. Also, if you are unable to run the program throughout the whole year, commit to a set number of weeks for each term.

The actual program will take a minimum of 16 minutes (five activity stations with three minutes on task time plus one minute combined changeover time) or a minimum of 26 minutes (five activity stations with five minutes on task time plus one minute combined changeover time) to complete, depending on the program running time chosen. However, do not forget about time for gathering children and sending them back to class, as well as time for setting up and packing away.

Due to different classroom demands or curriculum focus, at various times in your program planning or throughout the school year it may be necessary for you to combine two of the stations or even omit a station in order to fit the program into your class schedule and continue running it. Go ahead. The Fingergym™ program allows you to be as flexible with your program planning as you wish.

Helpful hint

- Look at your classroom schedule and decide when and how much time could be allocated for the program.

Who will run the program?

Will you, the teacher, run the program, or will you oversee and monitor it and have a trained teacher aide or volunteers run it? Involving teacher assistants, parents, grandparents, older student peers, or other interested community volunteers in the program may be a wonderful community builder.

Note. If your Fingergym™ program is to be run by a teacher aide or volunteer, your role will be to closely oversee and monitor the program, so constant communication and training is a must. Set aside a special Fingergym™ talk time in your schedule.

Helpful hints

- Determine who will be running and monitoring the program.
- Consider whether you would like to ask for volunteers to assist with the program. See the resource CD for a sample volunteer recruitment letter.

Where will the program be run?

Where the program will be run will depend on the program format chosen. Things to consider are:

- Do you have enough space in your classroom?
- Can you access a separate classroom or area for small groups or individuals?
- Is there enough room for storage of equipment nearby and easy access to this area?
- Can you leave the room set up or do you need to pack away after each session?

Helpful hint

- Think laterally about using 'free' or shared space within your school to set up the program.

How will equipment be accessed?

One does not necessarily need an extensive budget to start a fine motor program. There are a number of options to be considered here. Of course, if funding is available, look through catalogues and shops and spend up! If not, do not despair — try some of the following ideas:

- Begin your supplies collection with the purchase of five large storage containers. Large plastic see-through boxed on wheels are suggested as they are easy to store and transport.
- Use existing supplies — buy, recycle, beg, borrow, or do a deal.
- Look at the materials listed in each activity section in this manual. Run an inventory of existing classroom or toy-box materials, and think creatively.
- Raid your child's old toy boxes. Sometimes items considered to be outgrown and useless may serve a different purpose from their intended use, so re-invent an old toy's use.

- Use the class / parents' noticeboard to post a wish list of items that are needed (the recyclable-type things). For your inventory-keeping purposes, photocopy the supplies lists in each activity section in this manual and tick off each item as you get it.
- Shop at a discount store. These places are wonderful for 'gadgety' items and are usually so cheap — do try them.
- Recycle. Check out a recycling station — put on a 'think lateral or creative' hat and explore.
- For teachers who wish to order some unique Fingergym resources that are already made up, try our linked web site: www.fingergymresources.com

For additional information about accessing equipment, see also the Gathering and Sorting Equipment section.

Helpful hints

- Do you have money allocated in your classroom budget for supplies?
- Can this be a shared resource (for example, learning support budget)?
- Post a wish list of supplies to parents or other teachers once you have chosen your activities.
- Purchase five large plastic storage containers.
- Visit our linked web site (www.fingergymresources.com) for ready-made activities, materials and new ideas.

SETTING UP FOR THE PROGRAM

Choosing activities and preparing a schedule

For your convenience and to get you started, we have included a 24-session sample activity schedule on the resource CD. The activities included in this sample schedule have been chosen because of the availability of materials needed for them — either locally or through the Fingergym™ website (www.fingergym.info), the high motivational aspect and 'child appeal' of the tasks, and classroom suitability.

Of course, you may find it most beneficial to develop your own schedule using the activities and suggestions in this manual (see the blank activity schedule on the resource CD to get you started). Some advantages to choosing your own activities are:

- you can choose activities that use materials and equipment that you already have (especially if you do not have a big budget)
- your program can be tailored to meet the individual and special needs of your particular group of children.

Note. The activities in this manual progress from foundational strengthening activities, to sensory / planning and fine motor coordination activities, and then to more refined functional activities, such as pencil to paper and cutting.

Some general guidelines for choosing activities if you are developing your own activity schedule are:

Think big to small or foundational skills to applied skills. Keep in mind that starting with the larger and more global foundational activities, such as shoulder strengthening, before moving on to applied skills, such as handwriting or scissors work, is a good plan of action for implementing a fine motor program especially if you are running an individual program.

Choose activities that allow a measure of success. Start the program with an activity that the children can comfortably perform. If children have experienced repeated difficulty and failure with fine motor tasks, it will be very important to build up their confidence and skill level again. If an activity is too difficult and becomes frustrating for a child, for example, the child refuses to cooperate, scribbles, or avoids the task, consider adapting it to make it simpler, or choose a different activity all together.

Make sure that the task can be completed in the allotted time. Or, for a more complex craft activity, explain at the outset that this job may take two or three sessions to complete and that children should just get as much done as they can before the music starts. If an activity is taking more than one session to complete, set up a filing system for children to store their unfinished work in. Something easy to get at and within their reach is useful, as you will want to encourage the children to do this independently. A hanging shoe storer works well.

Consider the degree of supervision required for each activity. To make this easier, each activity has been categorised with a supervision level:

No or minimal supervision required

Some supervision required

One-to-one supervision required

The level of supervision required will also be determined by the specific needs of the children (not just physical but also intellectual, emotional, and safety issues) as well as the program format chosen.

Consider the number of available trainers. For example, if you only have one trainer and five children, you will probably be best to choose only one activity that requires one-to-one supervision. Alternatively, if you have four trainers, you could easily choose four activities that require one-to-one supervision. Similarly, if you are running the program with individual children or with a small group where the group rotates together, again you might be able to choose all activities that require a high level of supervision.

When covering a specific theme in class, such as underwater or space, choose or adapt activities that fit in with what the children are studying. For example, choose cutting and drawing activities of spaceships, planets, and so on. In this way, you can tie in fine motor activities with the academic curriculum.

Helpful hints

- Use the prepared 24-session activity schedule on the resource CD.

OR

- Develop an activity schedule using the blank activity schedule on the resource CD..

Gathering and sorting equipment

To run the Fingergym™ program, you will need the following items:

- five activity stations/tables
- CD player
- *Fingergyngles™* CD
- activity cards
- selected activity equipment, including worksheets and storage containers.

FIVE ACTIVITY STATIONS

Each activity station is used for one of the fine motor skills targeted in this program. These are strengthening skills, sensory and planning skills, fine motor coordination skills, pencil to paper skills, and cutting skills.

Set up activity stations either in the classroom or in a separate area. Consider the program format you are running when choosing where to set up the stations. For example, if running the program with individual children, it is best to set up the stations in a separate room so that they do not distract the other children in the class and the other children in the class do not distract them. Also, if you are running the program in small group rotation or whole class (small group rotation) formats, ensure that there is enough room at each station for all of the children in the small group to sit or stand around it. Other things to think about when setting up the activity stations are:

- You may choose to name the activity tables, such as the Strengthening Table or the Strong Hands Table.
- The table and chairs for the cutting and pencil skills stations need to be set up at correct work height. Tasks at other stations may require the children to stand to develop large muscle strength, or to use a large exercise ball as a chair. If the children are standing, ensure that the table is at the correct work height.
- Try to maintain the same set-up, with tables and stations in the same order each session, as knowing what is expected of them at each station helps children to settle more quickly to their activity.
- Remember, you can combine two of the stations or even omit a station if different classroom demands or curriculum focus at various times during the year conflict with running the Fingergym™ program in its entirety.

CD PLAYER AND FINGERGYNGLES™ CD

For additional information about the *Fingergyngles™* CD, see also the Using the *Fingergyngles™* CD section following. Remember that you will need to have a power point available for an electric CD player, or you will need a battery-operated CD player. Listen to the entire CD before you play it for the children, and choose the appropriate Fingergyngles™ track (running time) for your program. Remember, you can either run the program for 16 minutes or 26 minutes.

ACTIVITY CARDS

So that you always have a master copy of all activities in this program, it is recommended that you photocopy and laminate the activity cards that you have chosen for your activity schedule. You can then file these cards into a card-sized filing box according to their skills categories, such as strengthening activities (see example on resource CD). A benefit of this storage method is that you have quick access to the cards, as long as they are filed and re-filed in correct numerical order. Alternatively, you can place the laminated cards (you might even choose to enlarge them for easier reading) into their own snap-lock or resealable bag along with the supplies needed for that activity. Store these bags with others containing activities from the same skills section (for example, all strengthening activities would be placed into one large box) (see example on resource CD). The benefits of this storage method are that program trainers can go to one central place to get out both card and activity equipment, and it can also be handy on those 'fly by the seat of your pants' days when you need to quickly grab an activity.

ACTIVITY MATERIALS

Use the supplies lists in each activity section in this manual to identify what materials will be needed for your program. Supplies in the 'items from the common supplies box' lists are those that are common to other activities in different sections of the program. The supplies lists can be used to assist with gathering materials, either as a wish list that you can give to parents to ask if they could donate or contribute supplies, or just as an inventory as you purchase or gather equipment.

Note. Ensure that any recyclables that you are using are safe and clean.

Collect as much scrap paper of varying thicknesses and textures as you can find. Collect bubble wrap and cellophane, old holiday and birthday cards, wrapping paper, wallpaper scraps, magazines, and anything else you think may be perfect for the Fingergym™ program. Cut these materials into manageable sizes and store them in a clearly labelled box or bag. You will need lots of such materials.

As above, to ease the set-up process each time you run the program, organise a separate large box or plastic bag for materials needed for each skills section (for example, strengthening activities) and perhaps one large box for items that are common to many of the activities. Label these boxes and bags clearly, and include a supplies checklist and the corresponding activity card(s) and materials in the bag or box to help keep things in order. Volunteers might enjoy the fun and challenge of organising all of these boxes or bags.

From the resource CD, print out or photocopy any worksheets required for the activities and file these in clear plastic sheets in a large folder for easy access.

Also, parent information/permission slips, certificates and reward templates, some of which can be personalised, are also available on the resource CD. Print or photocopy and file these materials into folders or notebooks.

Helpful hints

- Plan the set-up of the five different activity stations according to the type of program format chosen.
- Check that you have a power point available if using an electric CD player, or have a battery-operated CD player.
- Choose the Fingergyngles™ track to be used (either 16 or 26 minutes).
- Prepare the activity cards for easy filing and access.
- Gather all equipment required, sort, and store it.
- Photocopy and file any necessary templates or worksheets.

TRAINING PROGRAM TRAINERS

Consider the training needed for volunteers and teacher aides who will be implementing the program. At this point in program planning, an occupational therapist will likely serve as a wonderful resource to give an in-service or even provide some initial training in fine motor development to staff and volunteers who will be involved with the program.

- Obtain some kind of commitment from program trainers, assuring that the 'show will go on'.
- Provide trainers with a copy of the Positive Fingergym™ Trainer and Trainers Mud Map information sheets found on the resource CD.
- Go through the general set-up of your program, including storage of materials, with your program trainers.
- Play the *Fingergyngles™* CD for the trainers.
- Encourage the trainers to have a go at and become familiar with the various activities that will be used in the program. Focus points are included on each card to assist with ensuring that the children are performing the activity in the correct manner. Highlight these to the trainers.

Helpful hints

- Set aside time for trainer training and feedback.
- Photocopy and distribute the Positive Fingergym™ Trainer and Trainers Mud Map information sheets to the trainers.
- Ask an occupational therapist to come and give an in-service on fine motor skills to the trainers.

RUNNING THE PROGRAM

Using the *Fingergyngles™* CD

The *Fingergyngles™* CD uses a musical cue to direct children to finish up at their current activity, move to the next activity, and begin the new one. In between each musical cue is silence, which indicates that the children are to work at their activity.

Step 1 Choose the appropriate Fingergyngles™ track (program running time). Track 1 has Fidget's™ and Mani's™ voice-over giving a brief explanation of how the program will run and instructions to ensure that the children are ready to start their first activity. You might want to use this track for the first few sessions until the children are familiar with how the program works. Track 2 allows for five 3 three-minute activities plus 15 seconds of changeover time between each activity (total program time = 16 minutes). Track 3 allows for five 3 five-minute activities plus 15 seconds of changeover time between each activity (total program time = 26 minutes).

Note. There is a three minute period of silence after Fidget's™ croak on Track 2 that should allow enough time to get to the CD player and turn it off before Track 3 begins.

Step 2 After the initial trainer greeting, simply turn on the CD

Step 3 Turn the CD off when you hear Fidget the Frog™ give a croak at the end of the final rotation.

Some suggestions for using the CD are as follows:

- For Session 1, choose Track 1 and then choose from Track 2 or Track 3.
- For subsequent sessions, choose Track 2 or Track 3.

Helpful hint

- Remember the format: no music = working time, music = changeover time.

Structure of the program sessions

The following instructions specifically apply to small out-of-class groups, but can be easily modified to suit in-class groups as well.

SESSION 1

- Bring the group of children who will be participating in the program to the special Fingergym™ room or area.
- Explain to the children why they are with you and what they are going to be doing in Fingergym™. Things that the trainer should try to make clear (the *Fingergyngles™* CD will also remind them about these things) are:
  - *Fingergym™ is going to be a fun time where you can practise making your fingers strong and clever.*
  - *There will be lots of different things to do but you will find one activity is based at each of these tables and must be done just there, so no wandering around please.*
  - *Some activities may need a bit of practice before you can do them really well, but there will always be help if you need it at Fingergym™.*
  - *Give things a go — even if an activity seems tricky one day, it will soon become easier with a bit of help and practice.*
  - *You only have a short time to do each activity, so you need to ask straight away if at any station you do not know what to do.*

- *Listen for the special Fingergyngles™ music. It tells you when to stop doing your activity and move on to the next one. You will not have much time to move, so listen carefully and move quickly to the next job.*
- *Try and remember to sit or stand up straight when you are working, so that your big body muscles get strong, too.*
- *Finally, remember to tidy up your place for the next person who will be doing the activity after you have finished.*

  Note. This instruction will be different if you are working with children who have difficulty getting started. These children will need to be encouraged to get to a certain stage in a job within a set time frame rather than be concerned with the clean-up part of the task.

- Explain what each activity requires using simple instructions, or, if an activity is self-explanatory and you want to encourage the children to ask for help, you may decide *not* to give specific instructions. Instead, the expectation will be for the children to quickly realise they do not know what to do and that they must raise their hand and ask for 'Help, please'.
- Give each child or group a starting activity. You may make one child the leader for the day. They can start at Station 1 (usually the strengthening station). A simple Fingergym™ leader badge or sticker may be very motivating (see the resource CD).
- Play Track 1 of the *Fingergyngles™* CD for an introduction, then play Track 2 or Track 3, depending on which one you have chosen.
- Assist the children to follow the program and rotate around the activity stations.
- When the program is finished, return the children to the main class area.

ALL SUBSEQUENT SESSIONS

- Give each child their starting position or allow them to choose one.
- Prompt them to gather their partially completed activities from previous sessions if necessary.
- Go over any specific activity directions.
- Begin the *Fingergyngles™* CD at the appropriate track.

Refer to the Tainers Mud Map on the resource CD for a quick guide to the session format.

Monitoring progress

Keeping track of each child's progress (especially in individual-based programs) is an important part of this program. The results can be helpful for teachers in that they can provide data for outcomes-based reports and can also assist in determining a profile of each child's fine motor strengths and weaknesses. From the classroom trials conducted with this program, teachers have also indicated that the Fingergym™ program has been useful for providing feedback about children's general readiness skills.

As teachers have busy assessment schedules, a Fingergym™ Program Progress Form (see resource CD) has been developed to assist with monitoring each child's progress in the program. The progress form is simple, quick, and easy to complete using three assessment criteria: S = satisfactory (activity was performed easily by the child), NI = needs improvement (activity was not easy for this child to perform), U = unable to perform activity (or unable to perform without modification). If you wish to also monitor progress with readiness behaviours, such as transitioning between activities, asking for help when required, and so on, a basic checklist for this has also been included on the resource CD.

If you are overseeing and monitoring but not directly involved in running the program, plan a set time into your schedule to meet with the program trainers to discuss the program and how the children are doing. You may choose to monitor progress by:

- completing a progress form after each session (This would realistically only be possible if you were running the program with an individual child or a very small group.)
- focusing on each child's progress at one particular activity station during a particular session
- recording one particular child's progress for an entire session at each activity station (Another program trainer would definitely be required on this day to assist with the general running of the program).

Helpful hint

- Remember that each activity card has focus points, which will help you to pinpoint specific areas to monitor.

READY, SET, GO CHECKLIST

This checklist has been designed to assist you to check that you have completed all of the set-up steps and are ready to run the program.

- ☐ Have I chosen the format in which I will run the program?
- ☐ Have I decided which children will participate in the program?
- ☐ Have I decided how often the program will be run?
- ☐ Have I decided who will run the program?
- ☐ Have I decided where the program will be run?
- ☐ Do I know how I will collect the materials needed to run the program?
- ☐ Have I decided which activities I will run?
- ☐ If applicable, have I drawn up my own activity schedule?
- ☐ Have I set up my activity cards and equipment, including any worksheets?
- ☐ If applicable, have I trained the volunteers and/or teacher aides who will be running the program?
- ☐ Have I determined which Fingergyngles™ track I will need to use?
- ☐ Have I familiarised myself with how to conduct each Fingergym™ session?
- ☐ Have I set up how to monitor the children's progress?

Section B
Fingergym™ Activities

This section contains over 140 activities. These activities are divided into five skills categories that support fine motor development: strengthening, sensory and planning, fine motor coordination, pencil to paper, and cutting. For ease of use, activities are presented in a reproducible card-style format containing information about the tools or items necessary to perform the task, simple directions to carry out the activity, and on most cards, how to change the activity to make it easier or harder, indicated by the icons ▽ and △.

For those of you who are interested in an integrated curriculum approach to fine motor skill development, **academic links** (ways to incorporate the activities in the curriculum) have been provided for all activities. These links include mathematics, science, laterality and directionality, language, reading, writing, and art. Links are noted by the icon 🔗.

To assist you in observing that the children are performing the activity correctly, **focus points** have also been included on each activity card. These are noted by the icon 🔍. These focus points are explained in greater detail at the beginning of each skills section. Copies of these more detailed explanations also appear in card format, for ease of reference.

Also indicated on each card is the **level of supervision** required for most children to perform the task. This is indicated by one, two, or three Fidget the Frog™ heads 🐸. To assist with planning, the activities are organised in order of amount of supervision required.

At the beginning of each skills section you will also find a **supplies list**, which can be photocopied and used as a wish list for obtaining or inventorying supplies.

Strengthening Skills

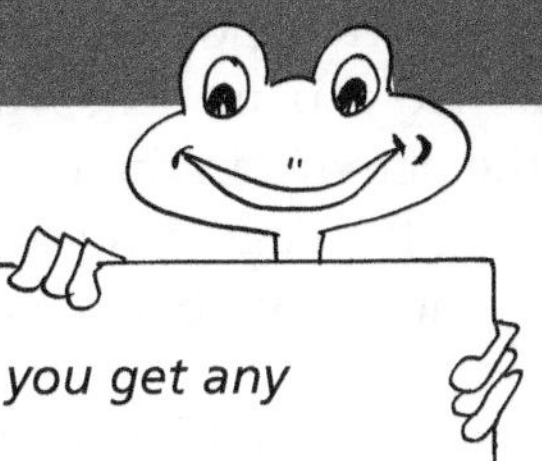

Teacher: *Please sit up straight James. Did you get any sleep last night?*

James always slumps at his desk and frequently holds his head in one hand. It is as though his spine just cannot keep him upright for more than a few minutes at a time. He frequently complains of a sore arm and fingers whenever writing work is introduced. James' work is often very sloppy and he complains of getting tired easily. His mother says he is just being lazy.

As outlined in Section A of this manual, muscles develop from head to toe and from the middle of the body outward. For example, shoulder and upper arm muscles develop before hand and finger muscles. This is a particularly important concept to understand because it means that to maximise fine motor function it is also very important to work with the 'big muscles' of the shoulders and arms.

Many children experiencing difficulty with fine motor activities may also have reduced muscle tone and strength in their trunk, shoulders, arms, and hands. Think of muscle tone as *tension*, the greater the tension, the more rigid something will be; the lower the tension, the more floppy it will be. Children with lower muscle tone and reduced hand strength often demonstrate loose wrist, knuckle, and finger joints. That is, it may look like these children have 'spaghetti hands'. The arches or curves of their hands may also be poorly developed so that their hands may appear flattened — lacking the bulge of muscles at the base of the thumb or on the other side of the hand under the little finger.

Children with lowered muscle tone and reduced strength may:

- tend to fatigue more quickly
- have difficulty maintaining good posture during floor time or when sitting at a desk
- complain of arm and hand pain during fine motor tasks
- have difficulty performing many tasks, such as writing, cutting, doing up buttons, pulling off socks and shoes, and opening lunch or food containers.

The activities in this section focus on strengthening the larger muscle groups of the body through Big Muscles activities as well as the smaller muscle groups of the hands through Strong Hands activities.

Strengthening activities focus points

When you are working on strengthening activities with the children, the following focus points will assist you in observing that they are strengthening the correct muscles and performing the activity in the correct manner. The relevant focus points can also be found in card format at the beginning of the Big Muscles and Strong Hands activity cards sections, for quick reference. A verbal cue or reminder for you to use is given for each focus point.

- **Bilateral coordination.** Ensure the children are using both sides of their body together in a smooth, coordinated manner. Ensure that both of their hands are being used together so that the dominant (worker) hand is performing the task and the non-dominant (helper) hand is stabilising or assisting. ***'Two hands'*** or ***'Where's the helper hand?'***
- **Crossing the midline of the body.** The midline is an imaginary line down the middle of the body. Ensure the children can cross their left leg/arm over to the right side of their body and vice versa without moving their whole body. ***'Body still, cross over'***
- **Finger isolation.** Ensure the children can move their fingers independently of each other. ***'Just your pointer finger'***
- **Hand dominance.** Take note of which hand each of the children generally uses. ***'Worker hand'***
- **Helper hand/worker hand.** The helper hand is the non-dominant hand and is used as a stabiliser or assistant. The worker hand is the dominant hand. ***'Helper hand/worker hand'***
- **Isolating movement.** Ensure the children can move parts of their body independently, such as their arms only. ***'Arms only'***
- **Level shoulders and shoulder stability.** Ensure the children's shoulders are even and not raised up to their ears. ***'Strong shoulders'*** or ***'Shoulders down'***
- **Maintaining position/sustaining grasp.** Ensure the children can hold or repeat a movement for a period of time, in order to build up endurance and strength. ***'Keep going'***
- **Patterning and sequencing.** Ensure the children maintain the rhythm, sequence, or pattern of movement. ***'Keep the pattern'***
- **Pincer grasp.** Ensure the children use the tip of their thumb and index finger. The space between the thumb and fingers should be open and in the shape of an 'O'. ***'Pinchy fingers'***
- **Planning and organisation.** Ensure the children have a plan to organise their movement or perform the task. Encourage them to think through the steps. ***'What's your plan?'***
- **Smooth, controlled movement.** Ensure movement is performed smoothly with no jerkiness or erratic movement at the beginning, mid-range, or the end. ***'Smooth moves'*** or ***'Steady hands'***
- **Thumb and finger joint stability.** Ensure the joints of the thumb and fingers are stable and not overly extended or wobbly. Encourage the children to ease off the pressure and try again. ***'Strong fingers'***
- **Tripod grasp.** Ensure the children use their thumb in opposition with their index and middle fingers. There should be an open space between the thumb and fingers. The ring and little fingers should be tucked away, closer to the palm. The middle finger joints should be bent. (see photo on page 78) ***'Pencil fingers'***
- **Visual tracking and focus.** Ensure the children can follow a moving object with just their eyes, without moving their head. Ensure they can keep their visual focus on a task. ***'Eyes on the job'***
- **Wrist extension and wrist stability.** Ensure the wrist is not bent in towards the body. It should be slightly extended. ***'Wrist up'***

☑ SUPPLIES LIST

For strengthening activities

Items from common supplies box

- ☐ Various types of paper
- ☐ Crayons, markers, pens, pencils, paint brushes, paints
- ☐ Tape
- ☐ Different-coloured chalk, chalkboard
- ☐ Shape, colour, letter, and number flash cards
- ☐ Towels
- ☐ Large ice-cream containers
- ☐ Boxes, tins, and containers
- ☐ Modelling clay
- ☐ Plasticine®
- ☐ Plastic clip-lock bags
- ☐ Plastic zip-lock bags
- ☐ Plastic spoons, ladles
- ☐ Paper cups and plates
- ☐ Pegs of varying sizes and resistance
- ☐ Small beads or treasures
- ☐ Play-Doh®
- ☐ Theraputty™
- ☐ Chenille sticks (pipe cleaners)
- ☐ String
- ☐ Sand
- ☐ Dried beans
- ☐ Glue
- ☐ Shoelaces

Additional items

- ☐ Rulers of varying types
- ☐ Scarves and gloves
- ☐ Small hoops
- ☐ Balloons
- ☐ Play Tunnel (available from toy stores, educational supplies catalogues, or some department stores)
- ☐ Balls
- ☐ Big stacking blocks
- ☐ Small trampoline
- ☐ Ropes
- ☐ Obstacle course items
- ☐ Suspended swing
- ☐ Small beanbags
- ☐ Quoits
- ☐ Wind-up toys
- ☐ Velcro® spots, tabs, or strips
- ☐ Collapsible animals
- ☐ Squeeze toys
- ☐ Various types of hole punches
- ☐ Various-sized rubber bands
- ☐ Pop beads or connector toys
- ☐ Toy hammers
- ☐ Styrofoam
- ☐ Golf tees
- ☐ Bubble wrap
- ☐ Plastic knives
- ☐ Spray bottles
- ☐ Squirt toys
- ☐ Circle target
- ☐ Bucket
- ☐ Timer
- ☐ Permanent marker
- ☐ Easels
- ☐ Spring binder clips
- ☐ Stickers
- ☐ Small gymnastics mats
- ☐ Scooter board
- ☐ Rolling pins, cookie cutters
- ☐ Tweezers, chopsticks
- ☐ Small plastic balls
- ☐ Masking tape
- ☐ Lap trays and biscuit trays
- ☐ Toy car
- ☐ Train tracks
- ☐ Cylindrical foam
- ☐ Blindfold

Strengthening Activities

Big Muscles

CARD 1

Strengthening (Big Muscles) Skills Focus Points

- **Bilateral coordination.** Ensure the children are using both sides of their body together in a smooth, coordinated manner. Ensure that both of their hands are being used together so that the dominant (worker) hand is performing the task and the non-dominant (helper) hand is stabilising or assisting. ***'Two hands'*** or ***'Where's the helper hand?'***
- **Crossing the midline of the body.** The midline is an imaginary line down the middle of the body. Ensure the children can cross their left leg/arm over to the right side of their body and vice versa without moving their whole body. ***'Body still, cross over'***
- **Finger isolation.** Ensure the children can move their fingers independently of each other. ***'Just your pointer finger'***
- **Hand dominance.** Take note of which hand each child generally uses. ***'Worker hand'***
- **Patterning and sequencing.** Ensure the children maintain the rhythm, sequence, or pattern of movement. ***'Keep the pattern'***

CARD 2

Strengthening (Big Muscles) Skills Focus Points

- **Helper hand/worker hand.** The helper hand is the non-dominant hand and is used as a stabiliser or assistant. The worker hand is the dominant hand. ***'Helper hand/worker hand'***
- **Isolating movement.** Ensure the children can move parts of their body independently, such as their arms only. ***'Arms only'***
- **Level shoulders and shoulder stability.** Ensure the shoulders are even and not raised up to the ears. ***'Strong shoulders'*** or ***'Shoulders down'***
- **Maintaining position/sustaining grasp.** Ensure the children can hold or repeat the movement for a period of time, to build up endurance and strength. ***'Keep going'***

CARD 3

Strengthening (Big Muscles) Skills Focus Points

- **Pincer grasp.** Ensure the children use the tip of their thumb and index finger. The space between the thumb and fingers should be open and in the shape of an 'O'. ***'Pinchy fingers'***
- **Planning and organisation.** Ensure the children have a plan to organise their movement or perform the task. Encourage them to think through the steps. ***'What's your plan?'***
- **Smooth, controlled movement.** Ensure movement is performed smoothly with no jerkiness or erratic movement at the beginning, mid-range, or the end. ***'Smooth moves'***

CARD 4

Strengthening (Big Muscles) Skills Focus Points

- **Thumb and finger joint stability.** Ensure the joints of the thumb and fingers are stable and not overly extended or wobbly. Encourage the children to ease off the pressure and try again. ***'Strong fingers'***
- **Tripod grasp.** Ensure the children use their thumb in opposition with their index and middle fingers. There should be an open space between the thumb and fingers. The ring and little fingers should be tucked away, closer to the palm. The middle finger joints should be bent. (see photo on page 78) ***'Pencil fingers'***
- **Visual tracking and focus.** Ensure the children can follow a moving object with just their eyes, without moving their head. Ensure they can keep their visual focus on a task. ***'Eyes on the job'***
- **Wrist extension and wrist stability.** Ensure the wrist is not bent in towards the body. It should be slightly extended. ***'Wrist up'***

BM1

Activity 1: Chair Push-Ups

Tools: Desk or table, desk chairs

Action: Children push their chair close to the desk and stand behind it with feet together about 20 cm from the back legs of the chair. Holding on to the backrest with extended arms, they move their body towards the chair by bending their elbows only and keeping their body straight, and then push out again.

△ Increase repetitions

Mathematics: Counting

Look out for children who compensate by bending their whole body into the chair rather than using just their arms; smooth, controlled movement

BM2

Activity 2: Easel Activities

Tools: Easels, paper taped to walls or doors, paints, brushes, crayons, markers, pens, pencils

Action: Children draw, trace, colour, or paint at an easel or on a vertical surface. This is helpful for developing mid-range control of the limbs when limbs are neither close to the body nor fully extended.

Art and Writing: Colour combinations, letter and number formation, planning, organisation of materials

Level shoulders/shoulder stability, wrist extension/stability, maintaining position over time, hand dominance, using whole painting area

BM3

Activity 3: Bottom Bumps

Tools: None

Action: Children lie on their back and then push up with their arms and legs so that only their bottom is touching the floor. They then lift their bottom up and lower it back down, and continue to repeat this.

△ Increase repetitions

Language and Mathematics: Counting (keep a time chart or graph or statistics for each child to monitor progress)

Shoulder stability; wrist stability; maintaining position; smooth, controlled movement

BM4

Activity 4: Bottoms Up

SEE PHOTO BM4 ON RESOURCE CD

Tools: Chair

Action: Children sit on a chair, with hands beside legs, and lift bottom/body off chair by pushing down through arms. Repeat.

△ Hold bottoms-up position for X seconds before releasing. Increase repetitions.

▽ Allow feet to remain on floor.

Mathematics: Counting (keep a time chart or graph or statistics for each child to monitor progress)

Shoulder stability, wrist stability, maintaining position

BM5

Activity 5: Crane Game

Tools: Paper, scarves, gloves

Action: Children lie on their backs and push up through their arms and legs so that their bottom is off the floor. Using their toes, they pick up objects such as crumpled paper, scarves, or gloves, and place them into a container placed to either side of their feet.

△ Use left leg to place objects into container located on their right side and vice versa.

Mathematics: Count the number of objects picked up each day (it may be fun to gather statistics and chart progress).

Shoulder stability; wrist stability; maintaining position; smooth, controlled movement, crossing midline

BM6

Activity 6: Balloon Volleyball

Tools: Balloons

Action: Children hit their balloon with their hands to keep it airborne.

△ Instruct the children to hit the balloon with specific fingers, wrist, elbow, or shoulder. Alternate hands or give a pattern to follow, such as left hand, left hand, right hand.

Mathematics: Keep track of the number of times each child can hit the balloon before it falls to the floor (it may be fun to gather statistics and chart progress).

Shoulder stability; wrist stability and extension; maintaining position; smooth, controlled movement; crossing midline; patterning

BM7

Activity 7: Chalk It Up

Tools: Different coloured chalk, chalkboard

Action: Provide children with a piece of different-coloured chalk for each hand, and ask them to start from the left side and draw simultaneous loops and waves across a vertically oriented chalkboard.

Mathematics and Laterality: Count the number of loops done each day (it may be fun to gather statistics and chart progress).

Hands should be apart, shoulders level and relaxed; wrist extension; tripod grasp; crossing midline; bilateral coordination

BM8

Activity 8: Hoop Spin

Tools: Small hoops (embroidery or commercially available gym hoops)

Action: Place a small hoop around each child's arm. To keep the hoop moving, the child must slowly rotate their shoulder.

△ Place a hoop on each arm and keep both hoops spinning at the same time.

Mathematics: Count how long children are able to keep the hoop moving and the number of repetitions done each day (it may be fun to gather statistics and chart progress).

Shoulder stability; wrist stability and extension; smooth, controlled movement

BM9

Activity 9: Big Blocks Stacking Games

Tools: Large blocks, containers, and boxes

Action: Children stack blocks, containers, and boxes of varying sizes to create towers and 'buildings'.

Mathematics: Count the number of blocks, measure how high the building is, organise blocks according to size

Smooth, controlled movement; shoulder and wrist stability; planning and organisational skills

BM10

Activity 10: Wall Push-Offs

SEE PHOTO BM10 ON RESOURCE CD

Tools: Wall, stickers or pre-made targets affixed to the wall

Action: Children stand with two feet together facing a wall, arms distance away, with their hands placed on the wall at shoulder height. They then bend their elbows and bring their face in towards the wall, ensuring that their body remains straight. For added fun, a target or sticker can be placed on the wall at nose height.

△ Place fingertips rather than palms on wall.

Mathematics: Count how long children are able to hold this position and the number of repetitions done each day (it may be fun to gather statistics and chart progress).

Smooth, controlled movement; shoulder and wrist stability; straight body

BM11

Activity 11: Trampoline Time

Tools: Small trampoline, balls, flash cards (optional)

Action: Children bounce on the trampoline. This is a great activity for enhancing muscle tone.

Hint: Children may enjoy having a mini 'jogger trampoline' to use in the classroom.

△ While bouncing, children recite nursery rhymes or the alphabet, count, list things in a category (such as animals, colours, and foods), say arithmetic tables, read flash cards, or catch different-sized balls.

Language and Mathematics: Recall/memory, categorising, spelling, counting

Smooth, controlled movement; visual tracking of the ball

BM12

Activity 12: Train Tunnel

Tools: Play Tunnel

Action: Children move through the tunnel in various ways, such as crawling, on their backs, on all fours, like a crab, or on their side.

△ Children find coloured spots, letters, numbers, or spelling words placed in the tunnel. Give each child numbers or letters to remember and then ask them to find them in the tunnel.

Language and Mathematics: Letter and number recognition, spelling, reading

Smooth, controlled movement; shoulder and wrist stability; planning and organisation

BM13

Activity 13: Body Table Game

SEE PHOTO BM13 ON RESOURCE CD

Tools: Balls, balloons, beanbags

Action: Children lie on their back, push up with their arms and legs so that their bottom is off the floor, and hold this position while trying to balance balls, beanbags, or balloons on their 'table' (stomach).

△ Increase the amount of time that the children are to stay in the table position. Children kick a ball to another child while maintaining the table position. Children recite numbers, number patterns, nursery rhymes, or the alphabet while in the table position.

▽ Allow bottoms to touch the floor and do small bottom lifts off the floor.

Language and Mathematics: Keep a time chart or graph or statistics for each child to monitor progress.

Shoulder stability, wrist stability, maintaining position

BM14

Activity 14: Obstacle Course

Tools: Chairs, tables, tunnels, blocks, small gymnastics mat, scooter board

Action: Children follow directions to complete an obstacle course of your design.

△ Increase complexity of course by adding more climbing, crawling, or movement challenges. Challenge memory skills by asking children to repeat instructions and then follow the course in the correct sequence.

▽ Decrease complexity of course by having fewer stations and simpler obstacles to conquer.

Language: Spatial directions (on/off, over/under, beside, between, behind, in front), temporal directions (after/before), and sequential memory skills

Smooth, controlled movement; planning and organisation

BM15

Activity 15: Wheelbarrow Walks

SEE PHOTO BM15 ON RESOURCE CD

Tools: Shape, colour, letter, and number flash cards (if desired)

Action: Children lie on their tummy and push up from the ground with their hands while a helper holds them at their knees and 'walks' them along.

△ Increase distance child walks. Have child lift one hand to reach for a 'treasure', such as a specified letter or number card placed at a height just off the floor or low on a wall.

▽ Hold children at the hips.

Mathematics: Count how long children are able to hold this position and measure distance walked.

Shoulder stability, wrist stability, maintaining position

Activity 16: Push and Pull Tug

BM16

Tools: Towels, ropes, scarves

Action: Child and helper stand, sit, or kneel opposite each other holding onto a towel at either end and play tug, or one child pulls on a towel or rope that is attached at one end to something stable.

Mathematics: Count the number of repetitions or 'wins' achieved each day (it may be fun to keep score).

Shoulder stability, wrist stability and extension, maintaining position

Activity 17: Push-Ups

BM17

Tools: None

Action: In order to protect growing joints, push-ups with knees on the ground are recommended for this age group.

△ Play 'traffic lights' by having children 'stop' and hold their position at various stages in the push-up and then 'go' when told to do so.

Mathematics: Count how long children are able to hold the push-up position and the number of repetitions done each day (it may be fun to gather statistics and chart progress).

Level shoulders; wrist stability; smooth, controlled movement

Activity 18: Row Your Boat

BM18

Tools: None

Action: With partners, children sit with legs stretched out in front touching their partner's feet and holding hands. Pairs pull and push each other as if rowing a boat. Sing *Row, Row, Row Your Boat*.

△ Have one partner pull the other up into a sitting position from a lying down position.

Language and Memory: Rhyming, verbal recall of song

Smooth, controlled movement

Activity 19: Swing High, Swing Low

BM19

Tools: Suspended swing, balls, beanbags, quoits, boxes

Action: Lying on their tummy on a bolster swing, children throw different items into a box, such as quoits and beanbags.

△ Specify items to be placed in different boxes, for example, different-coloured items or different types of flash cards (number, letter, or shape).

Mathematics and Language: Letter, number, colour, and shape identification

Shoulder stability, visual tracking, planning and organisation

BM20

Activity 20: Over the Line

Tools: Line drawn on ground, rope or string

Action: Child and partner kneel on either side of a line, join hands, and try to push each other over the line.

Mathematics: Score how many times each person can push the other over.

Shoulder stability, elbows should be slightly bent, wrist extension and stability

BM21

Activity 21: Body Drawing

Tools: None

Action: Children draw large circles in the air with their whole arm, hands, or fingers.

△ Draw letters or numbers or spelling words. Specify direction for circles to be drawn. Simultaneously draw with both arms in the same or opposite direction.

Mathematics, Laterality, Writing: Count the number of repetitions, left and right concepts, writing

Shoulder stability, maintaining position, isolating movements (such as holding shoulder and elbow steady while moving only wrist), hand dominance

BM22

Activity 22: Beanbag Toss

Tools: Towels, small beanbags

Action: With a partner doing the same, child takes two end corners of a towel. A beanbag is placed in the middle of the towel. Use the towel to toss up and catch the beanbag.

△ Children kneel while doing this activity.

Mathematics: Count how many repetitions the children do (it may be fun to gather statistics and chart progress).

Shoulder stability, maintaining position, visual tracking

BM23

Activity 23: Snakey Slides

Tools: Coloured paper; flash cards with shapes, letters, numbers, spelling words, or sight-word (if desired)

Action: Children slither like snakes across the floor, using their arms to pull themselves along the ground.

△ Place a sequence of flash cards with different colours, shapes, letters, numbers, sight words, or spelling words on them around the room, and have the children slither to them in the correct order.

Mathematics, Language, Reading: Sequencing, colour and shape identification, spelling and reading concepts

Shoulder stability, bilateral coordination, planning and organisation

Strengthening Activities

Strong Hands

CARD 1

Strengthening (Strong Hands) Skills Focus Points

- **Bilateral coordination**. Ensure the children are using both sides of their body together in a smooth, coordinated manner. Ensure that both of their hands are being used together so that the dominant (worker) hand is performing the task and the non-dominant (helper) hand is stabilising or assisting. ***'Two hands'*** or ***'Where's the helper hand?'***
- **Crossing the midline of the body**. The midline is an imaginary line down the middle of the body. Ensure the children can cross their left leg/arm over to the right side of their body and vice versa without moving their whole body. ***'Body still, cross over'***
- **Finger isolation**. Ensure the children can move their fingers independently of each other. ***'Just your pointer finger'***
- **Hand dominance**. Take note of which hand each child generally uses. ***'Worker hand'***

CARD 2

Strengthening (Strong Hands) Skills Focus Points

- **Helper hand/worker hand**. The helper hand is the non-dominant hand and is used as a stabiliser or assistant. The worker hand is the dominant hand. ***'Helper hand/ worker hand'***
- **Isolating movement**. Ensure the children can move parts of their body independently ,such as their arms only. ***'Arms only'***
- **Level shoulders and shoulder stability**. Ensure the shoulders are even and not raised up to the ears. ***'Strong shoulders'*** or ***'Shoulders down'***
- **Maintaining position/sustaining grasp**. Ensure the children can hold or repeat the movement for a period of time, to build up endurance and strength. ***'Keep going'***

CARD 3

Strengthening (Strong Hands) Skills Focus Points

- **Patterning and sequencing**. Ensure the children maintain the rhythm, sequence, or pattern of movement. ***'Keep the pattern'***
- **Pincer grasp**. Ensure the children use the tip of their thumb and index finger. The space between the thumb and fingers should be open and in the shape of an 'O'. ***'Pinchy fingers'***
- **Planning and organisation**. Ensure the children have a plan to organise their movement or perform the task. Encourage them to think through the steps. ***'What's your plan?'***
- **Smooth, controlled movement**. Ensure movement is performed smoothly with no jerkiness or erratic movement at the beginning, mid-range, or the end. ***'Smooth moves'***

CARD 4

Strengthening (Strong Hands) Skills Focus Points

- **Thumb and finger joint stability**. Ensure the joints of the thumb and fingers are stable and not overly extended or wobbly. Encourage the children to ease off the pressure and try again. ***'Strong fingers'***
- **Tripod grasp**. Ensure the children use their thumb in opposition with their index and middle fingers. There should be an open space between the thumb and fingers. The ring and little fingers should be tucked away, closer to the palm. The middle finger joints should be bent. (see photo on page 78) ***'Pencil fingers'***
- **Visual tracking and focus**. Ensure the children can follow a moving object with just their eyes, without moving their head. Ensure they can keep their visual focus on a task. ***'Eyes on the job'***
- **Wrist extension and wrist stability**. Ensure the wrist is not bent in towards the body. It should be slightly extended. ***'Wrist up'***

SH1

Activity 1: Play-Doh® or Modelling Clay Snakes

Tools: Modelling clay or Play-Doh®

Action: Children roll the modelling clay or Play-Doh® into a shape like a snake using both hands. They then poke their index finger along the snake, trying to keep the finger straight, and then pinch off small pieces of the 'snake' using only their thumb and index finger.

Mathematics and Language: Children keep track of how many snake pieces they make, colour identification (such as what colour snakes they made)

Encourage rolling with the fingers and not the base of the hand, finger joint stability, pincer grasp

SH2

Activity 2: Dinosaur Bones

SEE PHOTOS SH2 (PART 1) AND SH2 (PART 2) ON RESOURCE CD

Tools: Play-Doh® or modelling clay

Action: Place a golf ball–sized amount of Play-Doh® or clay in children's palms. Children must gently squeeze the Play-Doh® or clay through slightly opened, curled up fingers until it oozes between the spaces, and then slowly open the fingers one by one to reveal a 'dinosaur bone'.

△ Use firmer Plasticine® or Theraputty™ (a commercially available product)

▽ Use very soft Play-Doh® or soft Theraputty™

Mathematics and Language: Children keep track of how many bones they make; colour identification (such as what colour bones they made)

Finger isolation; smooth, controlled movement

SH3

Activity 3: Play-Doh® Cookies

Tools: Play-Doh®, rolling pins, cookie cutters

Action: Children use rolling pins and cookie cutters to make cookies or other bakery items out of Play-Doh®.

Language and Mathematics: Talk about how to make a recipe, sequencing, following instructions, dividing cookies into even groups

Wrist extension when rolling, encourage use of fingers rather than the whole hand when pushing down on cookie cutter

△ Give a set number of cookies to be made in the given time. Use smaller cookie cutters

▽ Use larger cookie cutters with a handle

SH4

Activity 4: Cutting Play-Doh® Sausages

Tools: Play-Doh®, plastic knives, rulers

Action: Children roll the Play-Doh® into a long sausage, then cut it with a plastic knife, ruler, or fingers

Hint: Increase supervision level if using a knife

△ Use firmer Plasticine® or Theraputty™

▽ Use very soft Play-Doh® or soft Theraputty™

Mathematics and Language: Children keep track of how many sausage segments they cut out or check whether they are the same sizes as the others or bigger or smaller than the others.

Hand dominance (make sure children are using the worker hand to cut and the helper hand to stabilise the object)

SH5

Activity 5: Clay Spiders

Tools: Modelling clay or Plasticine®

Action: While holding a clay ball in the palm of the helper/non-dominant hand, children use a pincer grasp (thumb and index finger tips) to pinch and pull the ball of clay to create spider legs.

△ Use firmer Plasticine® or Theraputty™

▽ Use very soft Play-Doh® or soft Theraputty™

Science, Language, Mathematics: Discuss spiders/insects, count number of legs

Finger isolation, pincer grasp, bilateral coordination

SH6

Activity 6: Play-Doh® Colour Mix Up

Tools: Play-Doh® (at least two colours), plastic zip-close bags

Action: Children put two or more chunks of different-coloured Play-Doh® in a zip-close bag and squeeze them together to make a new colour, using the pincer grasp.

△ Use firmer Plasticine® or Theraputty™

▽ Use very soft Play-Doh® or soft Theraputty™

Art and Language: Discuss colour combinations.

Pincer grasp, bilateral coordination

SH7

Activity 7: Peas Please

Tools: Play-Doh®, clay

Action: Children make pea-sized balls using just the thumb, index, and third fingers, then squeeze the peas and start again or stack them to make a tower.

Hint: Draw a circle 'race track' on the pad of children's thumbs to indicate the circular movements needed to make the pea.

△ Roll clay between thumb and index fingers only.

Mathematics and Problem-Solving: Incorporate counting and number games, such as 'Make three Play-Doh® nests with two eggs in each and then count how many there are all together'; do 1:1 correspondence (lay out seven pea-sized balls of clay or Play-Doh® and have children point to each as they count aloud)

Hand dominance, sustaining tripod or pincer grasp, wrist extension

SH8

Activity 8: Wind-Up Toys

Tools: Wind-up toys

Action: Children use thumb and index finger to turn the knobs on the toys.

△ Choose winding mechanism with greater resistance or smaller knob.

▽ Choose toy with a larger turning knob.

Mathematics and Directionality: Count how the toys move and in which directions they move.

Wrist extension, pincer grasp, isolation of wrist movement while rest of arm remains steady, hand dominance

SH9

Activity 9: Play-Doh® Treasures

Tools: Play-Doh® or clay, tiny objects such as beads of various shapes and small toy animals

Action: Children find the hidden object in the Play-Doh® or clay using only their thumb and index finger.

△ Use old and hardened Plasticine®. Children wear a blindfold. (Note: only blindfold children if they are comfortable with it.)

▽ Use very soft Play-Doh® and larger objects.

Language and Mathematics: Naming and categorisation of objects, counting objects

Hand dominance, sustaining a pincer grasp, wrist extension

SH10

Activity 10: Treasure Hunting

Tools: Sand in a cup, (collecting) container, small items, tweezers or chopsticks

Action: Using their dominant hand and a pair of tweezers or chopsticks, children dig around in the cup (held by their non-dominant hand) to pick out the tiny treasures and then place the treasures in another container (the collecting container).

△ Hold the cup above the table or at a point higher than the child's shoulder. Move the collecting container further from the child to prolong the sustaining of the pinching grasp. Children complete this activity while standing up.

▽ Rest or hold the container on the tabletop.

Language and Mathematics: Naming/categorisation of objects, counting

Hand dominance, shoulder stability, sustaining a pincer grasp

SH11

Activity 11: Collapsible Animals

SEE PHOTO SH11 ON RESOURCE CD

Tools: Plastic or wooden animals on a base with legs that collapse when a button underneath is squeezed

Action: Children hold their animal with their index and middle fingers on top of the base, with their thumbs underneath squeezing the button to make the animal move in different ways.

△ Isolate movements, such as make only the head or tail move. Use wooden animals as they are more resistant. Introduce left/right side concepts, such as make the animal's left side dance. Children hold the animal away from their body.

▽ Squeeze button fully to make the entire animal collapse.

Laterality and Directionality: Left and right, top and bottom

Sustaining movement, wrist extension, thumb movements, shoulder stability/level shoulders, bilateral coordination

SH12

Activity 12: Velcro® Pull-Apart

Tools: Velcro® spots, tabs, or strips; markers (if desired)

Action: Children use their fingers to pull apart or put together Velcro® spots, tabs, or strips.

△ Colour code or place letters, numbers, and/or shapes on the tabs. Following verbal or visual cues, children only pull apart specified tabs.

Mathematics and Language: Count the number of spots, time concepts (for example, how long it takes to pull tabs apart), and letter identification

Pincer grasp, bilateral coordination

SH13

Activity 13: Squeeze Toys

SEE PHOTO SH13 ON RESOURCE CD

Tools: Commercially available squeeze toys, small plastic balls, paper, masking tape, lap trays, toy car/train tracks, sand, biscuit trays

Action: Children use their fingers to squeeze the toy so that it blows small plastic balls or scrunched up paper around a pathway. Paths can be made with masking tape on a desk, a lap tray with a rim around it, an old car racetrack or train line, or made by the child in sand in a recycled biscuit tray.

△ Make paths more complex.

▽ No specific pathways.

Laterality and Mathematics: Go from left to right, count how long it takes children to navigate the balls or paper through the paths

Sustaining pincer or tripod grasp, visual focus, hand dominance

SH14

Activity 14: Bean Soup Exchange

Tools: Plastic spoons or ladles, paper cups, dried beans, cylindrical foam, children's own pencil grips (if desired)

Action: Each child receives a plastic spoon or small ladle and a paper cup of dried beans. They are to transfer the beans into a 'soup' pot placed in the centre of the table without dropping any off the spoon. The children are to hold the spoon in a tripod grasp (like holding a pencil).

▽ Build up the handle of the spoon using cylindrical foam or a pencil grip.

Mathematics: Count how many spoonfuls of beans it takes to fill the pot.

Shoulder and wrist stability; smooth, controlled movement; visual focus; tripod grasp; bilateral coordination; hand dominance

SH15

Activity 15: Magic Cutting

Tools: Newspaper or scrap paper, ruler, pen

Action: Children place a ruler on a piece of paper next to a line drawn on it, and use their helper hand to stabilise the ruler and paper while they use their worker hand in a pincer grip to tear the paper along the edge of the ruler.

△ Increase thickness or number of pieces of paper. Introduce corners for the children to tear around.

▽ Do not follow a specific line. Rule a thicker line.

Directionality and Mathematics: Concepts of top to bottom, count the strips

Bilateral coordination, pincer grasp on paper, hand dominance

SH16

Activity 16: Pop Beads and Connector Toys

Tools: Commercially available pop beads and connector toys

Action: Children use both hands to push beads and connector toys together and then pull them apart.

△ Children follow a sequence or pattern of verbal or visual cues.

Mathematics and Language: Sequencing and patterning, counting

Bilateral coordination, visual tracking and focus, planning and organisation

SH17

Activity 17: Hammering Games

Tools: Toy hammers, thick pieces of Styrofoam or similar material, golf tees

Action: Children press or hammer golf tees into a piece of Styrofoam or similar material to make a picture.

△ Attach Styrofoam onto a vertical surface to encourage wrist extension and strengthening. Instead of making their own picture, children copy a pattern or make a letter and/or number.

Mathematics and Language: Sequencing and patterning, number and letter concepts

Wrist extension when holding hammer, hand dominance

SH18

Activity 18: Bubble Wrap Pop

SEE PHOTO SH18 ON RESOURCE CD

Tools: Bubble plastic wrap, permanent marker, timer, coloured stickers

Action: Children pop large and small bubble wrap with fingers (pincer or tripod grasp).

△ Use fingers in a certain sequence, such as thumb and index finger, thumb and middle finger. Introduce a time to complete the activity, such as 'How many can you pop in one minute?'. Write numbers or letters on the bubbles with a permanent marker and have child pop only, for instance, the Bs or Ds. Place small coloured stickers or shapes on the bubbles for colour and shape discrimination.

Mathematics and Language: Counting; colour, shape, letter, and number recognition

Pincer and tripod grasp strength, hand dominance

SH19

Activity 19: Rubber Band Wrap

Tools: Various-sized rubber bands; various-sized jars, boxes, or containers

Action: Children place various-sized rubber bands around various-sized jars, boxes, or containers.

△ Use smaller and tighter bands that need more stretching. Have children follow a coloured sequence of bands.

Mathematics and Science: Problem-solving (what sized rubber band fits best on the jar?), counting, patterning

Bilateral coordination, sustaining grasp with open 'O'-shaped space between thumb and fingers

Activity 20: Paper Hole Punch Outs

SH20

Tools: Different-sized hole punches, paper, markers, glue

Action: Children use different-sized hole punches to create designs on paper. Encourage children to work out where the paper has to go to make the punches work.

Hint: Use punch out pieces in a collage, for a threading activity, or in a cutting activity.

△ Punch along a pre-drawn pattern with curves/angles. Use a more resistant hole punch. Use stiffer paper or thin cardboard. Introduce speed into the activity.

▽ Punch holes in a random fashion. Hold the paper for the child. Use lighter weight paper.

Mathematics and Art: Counting, patterning punch outs, collage

Thumb strength, bilateral coordination, hand dominance

Activity 21: Pegging: Tin-Top Patterns

SH21

Tools: Pegs, empty tin cans, rubber bands, spring binder clips

Action: Children place the pegs around the top of an empty can using a pincer grasp, and then remove the pegs by squeezing, not pulling.

△ Use more-resistant pegs or wrap rubber bands around the end of pegs to increase resistance. Introduce speed into the activity. Suspend the tin on its side.

▽ Allow child to use other fingers to assist with opening and closing the pegs.

Mathematics: Counting, patterning pegs

Sustaining a pincer grasp, wrist extension, bilateral coordination, hand dominance

Activity 22: Pegging: Hungry Crocs

SH22

Tools: Pegs; small items to be used as 'food'; small letter, number, or sight-word cards

Action: Children pretend pegs are crocodiles that are hungry to pick up 'food' (small items) in the 'water'. They lay pegs on their side and slide them along while pinching them open and closed with thumb and index finger.

△ Use more-resistant pegs. Give a time frame to complete the activity. Give a particular sequence of items to pick up.

▽ Allow child to use other fingers to assist with opening and closing the peg.

Language and Mathematics: Patterning, letter and number recognition

Sustaining a pincer grasp, wrist extension

Activity 23: Peg Match It

SH23

Tools: Pegs, word cards, sound symbol cards, number cards

Action: Children match word or other cards to a correct picture and peg them together with thumb and index finger.

△ Use more-resistant pegs. Give a time frame to complete the activity. Give a particular sequence of items.

▽ Allow children to use other fingers to assist with opening and closing the pegs.

Language and Mathematics: Patterning, letter and number recognition

Sustaining a pincer grasp, wrist extension, bilateral coordination

SH24

Activity 24: Peg Tight Rope

Tools: Pegs; string suspended like a tight rope; colour, shape, letter, number, and word flash cards

Action: Have children peg up colour, shape, letter, number, and word flash cards on a suspended string or wire with thumb and index finger.

△ Use more-resistant pegs. Give a time frame to complete the activity. Give a particular sequence of items.

▽ Allow children to use other fingers to assist with opening and closing the pegs.

Mathematics and Language: Counting; patterning and sequencing skills; colour, letter, and word identification

Shoulder stability, sustaining a pincer grasp, wrist extension, bilateral coordination

SH25

Activity 25: String Tug of Peace

Tools: String, shoelaces, chenille sticks

Action: Children grasp a piece of string or a chenille stick between their thumb and index finger, while a partner (helper) tugs on the other end. To be the winner, children are to try to get the middle of the string or chenille stick over a line.

▽ Use a thicker string or shoelace. Children use their whole hand.

Mathematics: Count how many wins the children have.

Sustaining pincer grasp, wrist extension, hand dominance

SH26

Activity 26: Target Practice

Tools: Spray bottles, squirt toys, circle target, bucket, balloons, string

Action: Children use spray bottles or squirt toys filled with water to hit a target, such as a suspended balloon, a target in a bucket, or a target drawn on the wall.

△ Use a smaller target. Make the target move. Children use just their thumb and index and middle fingers to squeeze.

▽ Use a stationary or larger target or no target.

Mathematics and Science: Measuring distance and pressure

Sustaining grasp, visual focus

Sensory and Planning Skills

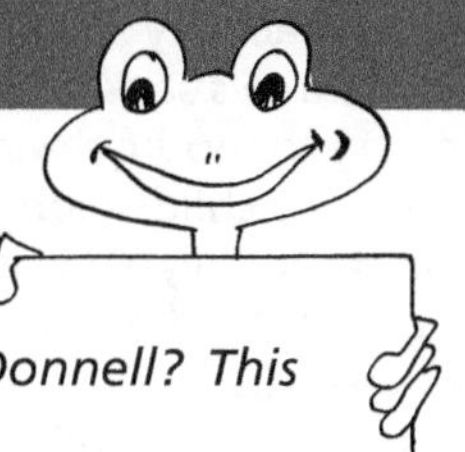

Jess: *Can I please wash my hands Mrs O' Donnell? This paint feels* really yucky *on my fingers!*

Teacher: *Soon Jess, but first let's look at your picture. Have you got all the right areas painted? — Where does the paintbrush go when you are finished?*

Jess is a 7-year-old who cannot stand having her fingers or feet in 'gooey stuff'. She also has trouble organising her work area, starting a task, and working out what to do, and frequently becomes easily distracted by outside noises.

THE SENSORY SYSTEM

The sensory system is a complex system, which includes the following parts:

- proprioceptive (joint position sense)
- tactile (touch awareness)
- kinaesthetic (sense of movement)
- vestibular (balance)
- auditory (hearing)
- visual (sight and perception)
- olfactory (smell).

When the parts of the sensory system are functioning in sync, they may be thought of as integrated (Ayres, 1979). A disturbance affecting one or more of the parts may have a negative impact on motor function, and even cognitive and perceptual skills. The effects of this may be seen in children's ability to plan and organise a new movement or a task, spatially organise their workspace so that their pencils do not keep rolling off the desk, or work out where to glue the picture so that it fits on the page.

How one interprets and ascribes meaning to what is seen, heard, or felt factors heavily into how we use our hands to write, cut, and manipulate objects as well as organise information and the environment around us. While the activities in this section focus largely on the tactile, proprioceptive, and kinaesthetic areas, many also focus on motor planning and spatial and sequential organisational skills.

Note. The activities within this sensory and planning section are multi-faceted and promote integration of the sensory–motor system.

IMPORTANT: It is critically important to monitor children when engaging in sensory activities. If a child expresses significant discomfort such as dizziness or nausea, remove them from the activity at once. However, if well tolerated, these activities will serve to enhance the children's sensory systems. If a child is reluctant to participate in the following activities, try to modify them. For example, instead of placing their hands in a tray of shaving foam, this child might enjoy squeezing the foam out of the can for their classmates. Then, gradually and gently reintroduce the child to a modified version of the task. If a child shows a defensive reaction to touching things, tolerance to tactile activities should be gradually increased at the child's pace. Keep in mind that formal sensory integration treatment is generally carried out in the clinic under the close supervision of a specially trained occupational or physical therapist. If you have questions or concerns about a child's sensory functioning, contact one of these therapists immediately.

KINAESTHESIA AND PROPRIOCEPTION: MOVE IT AND GROOVE IT ACTIVITIES

Some children seem to have a *need* to move in order to figure out where their body is in space and what it is doing. Sitting still at a desk in a classroom is perhaps one of the biggest challenges many of these children face. The inability to sit still can lead to the labels 'disruptive' or 'behaviour problem'. In the long term, self-esteem and thoughts about school and themselves as learners may also be negatively impacted by limited ability to remain still. While it can be very challenging to have these 'movers and groovers' in your class, some understanding and opportunities to incorporate their 'love of moving' into classroom life can make a positive difference for these children.

Helpful hints

- For children in your class who move constantly, fidget, get up from their chairs, and wander around the class disturbing others, offer short movement breaks at the 'power station' (see activity below) prior to sustained work time like handwriting lessons. For older students, the time in the power station could be used as an incentive or reward for focusing during specific lessons.
- You may also consider placing a lightly inflated travel cushion, or lightly inflated beach ball, or commercially available gel- or air-filled cushion on these children's seats, which allows for some wiggle movement without rocking the entire chair. Sitting on a large exercise ball for some lessons may also be helpful for some movers and groovers. Note: close supervision is required for this adaptation.
- Children who seem to constantly wander about the classroom may enjoy having a specific desk in a different part of the classroom to which they can go and work. To help with overall organisation, encourage these children to follow a specific route to get to this special desk.

Power Station

Tools: Bean bag chairs, kiddie pool, dried beans, foam blocks, 1 kg to 3 kg weights, large exercise balls, rocking chair, mini trampoline

Action: Create a power station, an area in which children may do one or a combination of the following:

- roll around on bean bag chairs
- do wall push-ups
- play in a kiddie pool filled with dried beans, foam blocks, or similar
- push boxes filled with objects of varying weights
- sit on large gym and exercise balls
- sit on a rocking chair
- jump on the trampoline.

FINE MOTOR PLANNING: HANDS AT WORK ACTIVITIES

Children demonstrating difficulty with fine motor coordination frequently have trouble organising their body movements, especially when faced with new motor challenges. Think of these challenges associated with carrying out novel hand and finger movements as fine motor planning difficulties. Weakness in fine motor planning may interfere with performance in cutting, drawing, and writing tasks as well as general organisation of work and handling of different materials and tools. There are a number of guidelines that may be helpful when working with children displaying fine motor planning difficulties:

1. Find out if the child has a 'plan' for performing the task. Ask the child, 'How do you do this job?'.
2. If the child does not have a plan, assist them to develop one. Before starting a task, encourage the child to visualise it in a step-by-step fashion.
3. Break the task down into easy steps — this is useful for identifying the problem area:
   (a) Work on an individual area of challenge by using a backward chaining method of instruction: child performs the final step of a task, then the last two steps, and so on, until the whole task has been learnt (Anderson, 2005; Turner, Lammi, Friesen, & Phelen, 2001). Or, try a forward chaining method in which the child performs the first step of a task, then the next two, and so on.
   (b) Encourage small successes to build self-esteem.
   (c) Encourage verbal rehearsal of the task: talk through the steps of an activity with the child and say the steps out loud. Eventually the child should be encouraged to whisper the steps quietly to themselves, and then to just say the steps in their head.
4. Use visual cues to assist with the planning of an activity, such as for correct finger placement on scissors or for a pencil grasp, or for where to point the scissors during cutting.
5. Coloured adhesive-backed paper can also be placed on the desk to assist with positioning of paper, pencils, and ruler.

SPATIAL AND SEQUENTIAL ORGANISATION: SEE, PLAN, AND DO ACTIVITIES

Another important aspect of performing classroom activities such as writing, cutting, setting work out on a page, or keeping a desk free of clutter is related to children's ability to organise themselves and materials in 'space' in an orderly and sequential manner (Levine, 2002). Hence, the child with difficulties in this area benefits from activities that require some planning and organisation of materials as well as provide opportunities to self-monitor and subsequently self-correct.

In this situation, it is important for the trainer to encourage the child to problem-solve and determine how parts of a puzzle go together, for example, where to place the rubber stamp so that it fits within the box, how to stack varying sizes of boxes so that they do not fall over, and so on.

All of these skills and many more assist the child in making a connection between what they perceive or 'take in', how they interpret that information, and how they do something purposeful with that information.

Sensory and planning activities focus points

When you are working on sensory and planning activities with children, the following focus points will assist you in observing that the children are performing the activities in the correct manner. These focus points can also be found in card format at the beginning of the Sensory and Planning activity cards section, for quick reference. A verbal cue or reminder for you to use is given at the end of each focus point.

- **Bilateral coordination**. Ensure the children are using both sides of their body together, in a smooth, coordinated manner. Ensure that both hands are being used together so that the dominant (worker) hand performs the task and the non-dominant (helper) hand stabilises or assists. **'Two hands'** or **'Where's the helper hand?'**

- **Crossing the midline of the body**. The midline is an imaginary line down the middle of the body. Ensure the children can cross their left leg/arm over to the right side of their body and vice versa without moving their whole body. **'Body still, cross over'**

- **Index finger isolation**. Ensure the children can move their fingers independently of each other. **'Just your pointer finger'**

- **Kinaesthetic awareness**. Ensure the children are aware of their body movements without relying on vision. Encourage them to 'feel' different movements. **'Eyes closed, feel the move'**

- **Memory**. Encourage the children to use their memory for touch, sound, or sight. **'Relax and remember'**

- **Patterning and sequencing**. Ensure the children maintain the rhythm, sequence, or pattern of movement. **'Keep the pattern'**

- **Pincer grasp**. Ensure the children use the tip of their thumb and index finger. The space between the thumb and fingers should be open and in the shape of an 'O'. **'Pinchy fingers'**

- **Planning and organisation**. Ensure the children have a plan to organise their movement or perform the task. Encourage them to think through the steps. **'What's your plan?'**

- **Self-monitoring**. Encourage the children to check their own work as they go and see if their plan is working. If not, encourage them to think about what they need to change or do differently. **'Does that look right?'** or **'Is your plan working?'**

- **Smooth, controlled movement**. Ensure movement is performed smoothly with no jerkiness or erratic movement at the beginning, mid-range, or the end. **'Smooth moves'**

- **Spatial awareness**. Ensure that the children are working within their own space both on their individual projects and when working with others, and also that they are aware of the position of objects being used in relation to each other. **'Mind the space'**

- **Tactile awareness**. Ensure that children are challenged but comfortable to experience different sensations with their hands. Gently reassure them if they are extra sensitive but do not force the children to touch things. **'Feel it'**

- **Timing of movement**. Ensure the children are aware of having their body and hand ready to perform a task. **'Hands ready'**

- **Tripod grasp**. Ensure the children use their thumb in opposition with their index and middle fingers. There should be an open space between the thumb and fingers. The ring and little fingers should be tucked away, closer to the palm. The middle finger joints should be bent. (see photo on page 78) **'Pencil fingers'**

- **Visual tracking and focus**. Ensure the children can follow a moving object with just their eyes, without moving their head. Ensure they can keep their visual focus on a task. **'Eyes on the job'**

- **Wrist extension and wrist stability**. Ensure the wrist is not bent in towards the body. It should be slightly extended. **'Wrist up'**

☑ SUPPLIES LIST

For sensory and planning activities

Items from common supplies box

- ☐ Various types of paper
- ☐ Crayons, markers, pens
- ☐ Pencils
- ☐ Chalk
- ☐ Sticky tape
- ☐ Baking tray
- ☐ Towels
- ☐ Plastic plates (varying sizes) with rim
- ☐ Balloons
- ☐ Perspex® sheet or folder
- ☐ Styrofoam trays
- ☐ Craft sticks, paddlepop sticks
- ☐ Glue
- ☐ String
- ☐ Paper clips
- ☐ Shaving foam
- ☐ Plastic clip-lock bags
- ☐ Plastic zip-lock bags
- ☐ Paint
- ☐ Marbles
- ☐ Tray with rim (e.g., Stable Table®)
- ☐ Play-Doh®
- ☐ Sand
- ☐ Scarf
- ☐ Shape, letter, number, colour flash cards
- ☐ Scissors
- ☐ Dried peas or lentils

Additional items

- ☐ Greeting cards, magazines
- ☐ Drinking straws
- ☐ Balls, targets
- ☐ Plastic rings
- ☐ Blindfold
- ☐ Lazy 8 template (see resource CD)
- ☐ Dry rice, wheat, salt
- ☐ Bowl or empty ice-cream container
- ☐ Water snakes (commercially available)
- ☐ Magnets, washers
- ☐ Paddleball toy
- ☐ Eyedroppers
- ☐ Porous paper, blotting paper, or coffee filters
- ☐ Puzzles (store bought or homemade from greeting cards)
- ☐ Magnetic wheel (commercially available)
- ☐ Magnetic fishing game (homemade or store bought)
- ☐ Plastic or wooden race tracks
- ☐ Mazes
- ☐ Small toy cars
- ☐ Small blocks, LEGO®, K'NEX®
- ☐ Nesting boxes or cups
- ☐ Writing Line Cat Stamp (available from www.fingergym.resources.com)
- ☐ Stacking blocks of two different colours
- ☐ Coloured rubber bands
- ☐ Sandpaper
- ☐ Hand lotion (hypoallergenic)
- ☐ Tactile cards (homemade or store bought)
- ☐ Carpet squares
- ☐ Finger puppets
- ☐ Fidget Frog™ bendy toy (available from www.fingergym.info)
- ☐ Fidget™ plays 'can you copy me?' cards (available from www.fingergym.resources.com)
- ☐ Stamp in line perspex® animal stamps (available from www.fingergym.resources.com)
- ☐ Inkpad
- ☐ Sponge (household)
- ☐ Foam- or plastic-coated bendable wire animals (commercially available)
- ☐ Chenille sticks (pipe cleaners)
- ☐ Rice, wheat, sand, salt, popcorn kernels
- ☐ Coins, keys, number and letter magnets, shape blocks
- ☐ Bottles

Sensory and Planning Activities

CARD 1

Sensory and Planning Skills Focus Points

- **Bilateral coordination**. Ensure the children are using both sides of their body together, in a smooth, coordinated manner. Ensure that both hands are being used together so that the dominant (worker) hand performs the task and the non-dominant (helper) hand stabilises or assists. **'Two hands'** or **'Where's the helper hand?'**
- **Crossing the midline of the body**. The midline is an imaginary line down the middle of the body. Ensure the children can cross their left leg/arm over to the right side of their body and vice versa without moving their whole body. **'Body still, cross over'**
- **Index finger isolation**. Ensure the children can move their fingers independently of each other. **'Just your pointer finger'**
- **Kinaesthetic awareness**. Ensure the children are aware of their body movements (without relying on vision). Encourage them to 'feel' different movements. **'Eyes closed, feel the move'**

CARD 2

Sensory and Planning Skills Focus Points

- **Memory**. Encourage the children to use their memory for touch, sound, or sight. **'Relax and remember'**
- **Patterning and sequencing**. Ensure the children maintain the rhythm, sequence, or pattern of movement. **'Keep the pattern'**
- **Pincer grasp**. Ensure the children use the tip of their thumb and index finger. The space between the thumb and fingers should be open and in the shape of an 'O'. **'Pinchy fingers'**
- **Planning and organisation**. Ensure the children have a plan to organise their movement or perform the task. Encourage them to think through the steps. **'What's your plan?'**
- **Self-monitoring**. Encourage the children to check their own work as they go and see if their plan is working. If not, encourage them to think about what they need to change or do differently. **'Does that look right?'** or **'Is your plan working?'**

CARD 3

Sensory and Planning Skills Focus Points

- **Smooth, controlled movement**. Ensure movement is performed smoothly with no jerkiness or erratic movement at the beginning, mid-range, or the end. **'Smooth moves'**
- **Spatial awareness**. Ensure that the children are working within their own space both on their individual projects and when working with others, and also that they are aware of the position of objects being used in relation to each other. **'Mind the space'**
- **Tactile awareness**. Ensure the children are challenged but comfortable to experience different sensations with their hands. Gently reassure them if they are extra sensitive. **'Feel it'**
- **Timing of movement**. Ensure the children are aware of having their body and hand 'ready' to perform a task. **'Hands ready'**

CARD 4

Sensory and Planning Skills Focus Points

- **Tripod grasp**. Ensure the children use their thumb in opposition with their index and middle fingers. There should be an open space between the thumb and fingers. The ring and little fingers should be tucked away, closer to the palm. The middle finger joints should be bent. **'Pencil fingers'**
- **Visual tracking and focus**. Ensure the children can follow a moving object with just their eyes, without moving their head. Ensure they can keep their visual focus on a task. **'Eyes on the job'**
- **Wrist extension and wrist stability**. Ensure the wrist is not bent towards the body. It should be slightly extended. **'Wrist up'**

SP1

Activity 1: Rice and Wheat Play

Tools: Rice, wheat, sand, or salt; popcorn kernels, coins, keys, number and letter magnets, shape blocks; bowl; bottles (optional)

Action: Children are to find hidden objects in a bowl of rice, wheat, or similar.

△ Have children transfer rice, wheat, or similar through the opening of a bottle using their hands as a funnel. Blindfold children or cover their hands and have them describe, draw, or write the name of the hidden object. Place identical items in a row in front of the children and have them point to or feel for the item that is the same as the one in their hand.

Language and Writing: Object and letter identification

Tactile awareness, kinaesthetic awareness, memory

SP2

Activity 2: Sand Play

Tools: Sand, cups, Styrofoam or baking tray, water, toy cars

Action: Place a cup or two of sand onto an empty Styrofoam or baking tray. Children make pathways and patterns in the sand with their index finger, or make toy cars follow a path.

Hint: For fun and variety, consider using fish tank sand as it is available in different colours.

△ Use wet and dry sand combination. Present a pattern placed in a vertical orientation in front of the children and have them copy it in the sand tray.

Writing and Mathematics: Drawing letters, numbers, and shapes; weighing out and measuring the amount of sand used for this activity

Tactile and kinaesthetic awareness, index finger isolation, planning skills

SP3

Activity 3: Water Snakes

SEE PHOTO SP3 ON RESOURCE CD

Tools: Commercially available water snakes (slippery, coloured plastic tubes filled with water).

Action: In standing position, children transfer the water snake from their dominant hand (on top) to their other hand by gently squeezing it out of the upper hand and quickly catching it with the lower.

△ Stand away from the table and increase the distance between the hands.

▽ Do activity over a tabletop so children can rest their lower hand on the table.

Mathematics and Organisation: Count the number of catches

Tactile awareness, visual focus, planning, timing of movement, spatial awareness

SP4

Activity 4: Dancing Magnets

Tools: Magnets; small baking trays; washers, paper clips, other small metal items

Action: Using a magnet and a metal surface such as a baking tray, children manoeuvre a metal object around the surface by grasping a magnet beneath the tray with their dominant hand. The helper hand holds the tray steady.

△ Draw a pathway, maze, or letters and numbers for the magnet or metal object to travel around and through.

▽ Suspend the tray on two books or containers, leaving the middle section free.

Laterality and Language: Top and bottom, right and left; number concepts

Bilateral coordination, spatial awareness, visual tracking, planning and organisation

SP5

Activity 5: Paddleball Game

Tools: Commercial paddleball toy

Action: Children hit a small ball attached to a wooden paddle or bat via a piece of elastic cord.

Mathematics: Count the number of repetitions done each day (it may be fun to gather statistics and chart progress).

Visual tracking and focus; timing of movement; smooth, controlled movement; wrist extension; planning and organisation

SP6

Activity 6: Nesting Boxes

Tools: Gift boxes of various sizes, nesting cups or boxes, blindfold

Action: Children arrange gift boxes of various sizes or nesting cups or boxes in the right order to properly nest.

△ Have children make a tower with the boxes. Children wear a blind-fold and sort by feel (Note: only blindfold children if they are comfortable with it). Sort boxes with corresponding lids if available.

▽ Use only a few boxes with more obvious differences in their size.

Laterality and Directionality: Size concepts; top and bottom, right and left concepts; spatial concepts

Bilateral coordination, planning and organisation, spatial awareness

SP7

Activity 7: Eye-Dropper Game

Tools: Eye-dropper, paint, porous paper such as coffee filters

Action: Children fill eye-dropper with paint and squeeze with their fingers to drip it onto porous paper to achieve a tie-dye effect. Encourage children to cover all of the paper.

△ Use a more resistant eye dropper. Or outline a specific area to be coloured in specific paint colours.

Science and Mathematics: Early concepts of area and absorption

Pressure awareness, such as how hard to squeeze; pincer grasp; planning and organisation; self-monitoring; kinaesthetic awareness; spatial awareness

SP8

Activity 8: String Follow

Tools: Glue, paper, string, scarf, blindfold

Action: Glue string onto a page and have children trace over the pattern with their index and other fingers. Children lose a point if their finger slips off the path into the 'mud', or gain five points if they reach the end without 'falling off'.

△ Vary fingers used to trace along pattern. Do this with eyes blind-folded or hands covered with a light scarf or sheet of paper. (Note: only blindfold children if they are comfortable with it.)

Laterality and Directionality: Turning in different directions to trace the pattern

Finger isolation, tactile awareness, kinaesthetic awareness, spatial awareness

SP9

Activity 9: Magnetic Wheel

SEE PHOTO SP9 ON RESOURCE CD

Tools: Magnetic wheel (a commercially available toy)

Action: Children hold the magnetic wheel at arms length from the body, and by tilting their hand at the wrist make the wheel travel along its path.

△ Hold the device out and at shoulder height to increase shoulder strength and stability. Use non-dominant hand, or one wheel in each hand.

▽ Hold the wheel closer to the body and lower the arm to waist height.

Mathematics and Science: Keep track of how long the wheel travels on the path, concepts of motion and gravity

Shoulder and wrist stability, planning and organisation, visual tracking, kinaesthetic awareness

SP10

Activity 10: Marble Racing

Tools: Marbles, rimmed plastic plate, lap tray with outer groove (e.g., Stable Table®), sponge (if required)

Action: Children stand, hold the plate/tray out in front of them at chest height, and make small rotating movements with their hands and wrists to make the marble move around the inner edge of the plate or in the groove of the tray.

△ Change direction. Add a second and third marble.

▽ Rest tray or plate on a sponge on the desk, or directly on the desk.

Mathematics: Count or time number of rotations completed

Planning and organisation; smooth, controlled movement; shoulder and wrist stability; visual tracking; spatial awareness

SP11

Activity 11: Puzzle Mania

Tools: Puzzles, magazines, greeting cards, scissors

Action: Offer children a variety of puzzles ranging from simple inset puzzles for younger children to more complex interlocking puzzles for older children.

Tip: Make your own puzzles by cutting up pictures in a magazine or old greeting cards. Children can cut a picture into simple pieces and then arrange them again to make the complete picture.

Mathematics: Spatial concepts

Planning and organisation, self-monitoring, spatial awareness

SP12

Activity 12: Magnetic Fishing Game

Tools: Stick, string, magnet, container, metal pieces, letter/number flash cards, glue

Action: Children 'fish' with magnetic fishing rod and metal pieces.

△ Fish out letter from container to match the sound given, or similarly, use 'fishing' principle for number, addition, subtraction, and spelling activities.

▽ Use larger pieces of metal or a larger magnet. Use a larger rod.

Mathematics and Language: Sequencing and patterning, memory, number and letter concepts

Planning and organisation, shoulder and wrist stability, visual focus, kinaesthetic awareness

SP13

Activity 13: Race Track

Tools: Plastic or wooden tracks, mazes, pencils, small cars

Action: Trace around plastic or wooden tracks or mazes using fingers, pencils, small cars.

△ Increase resistance by making tracks in Play-Doh® or wet sand.

▽ Widen the path and use fewer curves.

Laterality and Directionality: Turning in different directions to navigate the maze

Planning and organisation, visual tracking, tactile awareness, spatial awareness

SP14

Activity 14: Writing Line Cat Stamp

Tools: Cat Stamp, paper, pencils

Action: Use the Cat Stamp to increase children's awareness of the writing lines and spacing between words appropriate to their year level. Encourage slow and deliberate stamping between the writing lines.

Hint: Encourage stamp — space — stamp — space, from left to right.

△ Make the cat's whiskers touch each other on the lines.

▽ Give a visual cue as to where the stamps should go, such as a small mark on the line.

Handwriting: Spatial orientation

Planning and organisation, self-monitoring, tripod grasp on stamp, visual focus, spatial awareness, tactile awareness

SP15

Activity 15: Marble Blow

Tools: Marbles, drinking straws, plastic plate or lap tray with a trough around the outer edge (e.g., Stable Table®), sand

Action: Using a straw, children blow a marble around a track made in clean, fine, white sand or around the outer trough of a lap tray.

△ Children hold the tray at chest height while blowing the marble around the track.

▽ Use a lighter marble for easier blowing.

Science, Laterality, Directionality: Concepts of motion and velocity; left and right, top and bottom concepts

Visual tracking, lip movement, planning and organisation

SP16

Activity 16: Stack 'Em Up

Tools: Stackable objects such as cups and blocks or stacking pegs

Action: Place two different-coloured stacking objects on either side of the children's midline, for example, red to the left, blue to the right. The children alternately stack objects to make a striped effect.

△ Use opposite hand to collect from each side (left hand crosses midline to pick up from the right side and vice versa). Children close eyes while stacking the cups or blocks, then check at the end if they have the right striped pattern.

Laterality and Language: Right and left, colour identification

Kinaesthetic awareness, bilateral coordination, sequencing, crossing midline, spatial awareness

SP17

Activity 17: Lazy Eights in the Rice

SEE PHOTO SP17 ON RESOURCE CD

Tools: Rice, sand, pebbles/gravel, peas or lentils; lazy 8 template; baking tray

Action: Children practise drawing lazy eights with the index finger of their dominant hand. Make sure that the tray or container of rice or other textured items is directly in front of the child so that they cross their midline when drawing. Provide the lazy 8 template for them to copy.

△ Children close their eyes.

Writing: Pre-writing skills

Finger isolation, crossing the midline, planning and organisation, tactile awareness, kinaesthetic awareness

SP18

Activity 18: Ball Games

Tools: Balls, targets, large balloons

Action: Ball play that includes catching, bouncing, throwing into the air and catching, dribbling, throwing at a target on a wall or floor, and/or juggling.

△ Use a smaller ball and target, use one hand, clap in between catches, and/or increase distance between partners.

▽ Decrease the distance between partners. Use a large ball or inflated balloon, which provides increased time for child to respond and visually track it.

Mathematics: Count repetitions (it may be fun to gather statistics and chart progress)

Visual focus/tracking, planning and organisation, timing of movement, spatial awareness, self-monitoring, bilateral coordination

SP19

Activity 19: Hand-Clapping Games

Tools: Rubber bands, plastic rings, finger puppets

Action: Children place their hands together with palms touching, and then clap individual fingers together several times and then all fingers together. Lead children through a series of fun finger-clapping combinations.

Hint: Place coloured rubber bands, different rings, or finger puppets on fingers to make this more exciting.

△ Give a finger sequence that children have to remember and gradually increase the length of the sequence.

Language, Mathematics, Memory: Sequencing skills

Finger isolation, motor planning, sequencing, visual focus, spatial awareness, tactile awareness, kinaesthetic awareness

Activity 20: Sticky Fingers

SP20

Tools: Sticky tape

Action: Wrap sticky tape around children's fingers a couple of times. Children remove the tape with other fingers on the same hand. Remove tape first from index finger, then from the middle, ring, and pinky fingers. This is also a great finger strengthening activity.

▽ Remove tape with fingers of other hand.

Mathematics: Sequencing

Tactile awareness, finger manipulation, finger strength, kinaesthetic awareness, planning and organisation

Activity 21: Smooth Shave

SP21

Tools: Shaving foam, Styrofoam trays or silver baking tray, container of water and towel, lazy 8 template

Action: Children draw different patterns including lazy eights in the shaving foam after spreading it over the whole tray.

Hint: Be sure to have a container of water and towel for clean up.

△ Children close eyes and draw different nominated shapes, letters, or numbers in the tray of shaving foam. Show a pattern to be copied and then remove it to encourage memory skills.

Writing: Pre-writing; copying skills; letter, number, shape formation

Tactile awareness, planning and organisation, memory , kinaesthetic awareness, crossing the midline

Activity 22: Rough and Write

SP22

Tools: Sandpaper letters/numbers; green and red pen; pens, crayons, or pencils

Action: Cut large letters or numbers out of coarse sandpaper for the children to trace over with their fingers and pencils. Place a green dot at the start point and a red dot at the stop point. Encourage the children to verbalise the 'letter story' (that is, how it formed) while they trace it.

Hint: Trainers can check with the classroom teacher for letter stories or specific words that they use to teach letter formation.

△ Draw the letter in the air afterwards to reinforce the motor memory pattern for the letter.

Writing and Language: Letter formation

Tactile awareness, planning and organisation, memory, spatial awareness

Activity 23: Finger Paint

SP23

Tools: Paint, salt, shaving foam, Styrofoam trays, paper, container of water and towel

Action: Finger paint using paint mixed with salt crystals or shaving foam. Encourage children to use different parts of their hand and fingers to make various patterns.

Hint: Be sure to have a container of water and towel for clean up.

Writing and Art: Write letters, words, or just create an original masterpiece

Tactile awareness, finger isolation, planning and organisation, using the whole page, spatial awareness

Activity 24: Tactile Cards

SP24

Tools: Two sets of cards with matching tactile surfaces (handmade or commercially available), blindfold

Action: Create a double deck of cards with different textures and 3-D shapes on them. While blindfolded, children identify similar textures and/or shapes.

Language: Object identification

Tactile awareness, memory, planning and organisation

Activity 25: Hand Lotion Fun

SP25

Tools: Hypoallergenic lotion

Action: Place a small dab of low scent hypoallergenic hand lotion on children's hands. Children rub both hands together, using either slow or brisk movements.

Laterality and Directionality: Rub fingers of right hand, rub thumb and pinky of left hand, right hand rubs on top of left hand, rub hands together above the head, rub hands together down towards the floor, and so forth

Tactile awareness, kinaesthetic awareness, planning and organisation

Activity 26: Shave the Balloon

SP26

Tools: Shaving foam, balloons, craft sticks, container of water and towel

Action: Children squeeze out and spread shaving foam on an inflated balloon. Give children a craft stick and ask them to 'shave' the balloon. To increase the sensory feedback, have them use their hand instead of a stick.

Hint: Be sure to have a container of water and towel for clean up.

Laterality and Directionality: Shave on top of balloon and on the front and back

Tactile awareness, planning and organisation ('Is the entire balloon covered or shaved?'), bilateral coordination

Activity 27: Shaving Foam Colour Change

SP27

Tools: Shaving foam, thick paint, zip-top resealable bag, towel and container of water

Action: Squirt a small amount of foam inside the bag. Add a glob of thick paint then seal the bag tightly. Children use a pincer grasp to mix the paint into the foam until no white foam is showing.

Hint: Be sure to have a container of water and towel for clean up

△ Use the pinching fingers of both hands.

▽ Use only the dominant hand.

Art: Colour mixing

Tactile awareness, pincer grasp, planning and organisation ('Is all the foam coloured?')

SP28

Activity 28: Carpet Creations

Tools: Carpet squares, chalk

Action: Children draw letters, numbers, or shapes with chalk on an old carpet square, and then erase their work with hands or fingers. Using chalk on carpet squares provides a bit of extra resistance and also offers children a different sensory experience.

Hint: Be aware of children with dust allergies.

△ Copy figures from the vertical plane to the horizontal.

Handwriting and Mathematics: Stress correct letter and number formation, copying skills

Tripod grasp, tactile awareness, kinaesthetic awareness, memory, letter/number formation, spatial awareness

SP29

Activity 29: Stamp in Line

Tools: Various stamps (see supplies list), inkpad, ruled and plain paper

Action: Children make a row of stamps to fit inside two ruled lines. Encourage children to apply even pressure.

Hint: Use clear perspex® or plastic stamp blocks. This allows children to check the alignment before stamping.

△ Use smaller stamps and narrow lines. Incorporate a sorting and patterning activity by using two or more stamps.

▽ Use large stamps and wide lines or no lines to begin with.

Mathematics, Laterality, Directionality: Counting, categorising, patterning

Tripod grasp, planning and organisation, self-monitoring, spatial awareness

SP30

Activity 30: Bendy Animals

SEE PHOTO SP30 ON RESOURCE CD

Tools: Commercially available foam- or plastic-coated bendable wire animals, such as bunnies, frogs, or monkeys, or chenille sticks

Action: Trainers bends the animals into a specific position. Children look at the model and try to manipulate the bendable toy into that shape.

△ Make the positions more intricate.

▽ Simplify positions and/or try using chenille sticks instead of bendy animals.

Language, Laterality, Directionality: Body parts orientation, left and right and top and bottom concepts

Planning and organisation, orientation of body parts, copying skills, self-monitoring, manipulation

SP31

Activity 31: Copy Fidget™

SEE PHOTO SP31ON RESOURCE CD

Tools: Fidget Frog™ bendy toys, 'copy me' cards

Action: Place card in vertical position in front of the children. Children manipulate Fidget Frog™ to look the same as the card. Encourage children to check for accuracy by placing Fidget™ on top of the card. Continue this process until accuracy is achieved.

△ Use more difficult cards. Introduce 3-D positions or more than one frog.

▽ Place card flat on the desk. Children place Fidget™ directly on top of card.

Language and Directionality Concepts: Left/right, up/down, curved/straight

Planning and organisation, orientation of body parts to each other, spatial awareness, copying skills, self-monitoring, manipulation

Activity 32: Finger-Pattern Sequences

SP32

SEE PHOTO SP32 ON RESOURCE CD

Tools: Marker pen

Action: Number each finger on children's hands, starting with the thumb (1). Children copy a finger pattern such as (1–4): thumb (1) touches ring finger (4).

△ Model a sequence of finger patterns to be remembered, such as thumb to 2, 5, 4. Increase number of repetitions of the pattern. Replace numbers with letters and children spell out words.

Language and Mathematics: Finger identification, spelling skills, memory skills, finger and number correspondence concepts

Finger awareness, using tips of fingers, planning and organisation, memory

Activity 33: Chalk Artists

SP33

Tools: Chalk, cemented area

Action: Children draw on playground asphalt or other cemented areas. This activity is great to increase sensory feedback when learning to write letters and numbers.

△ Use thin pieces of chalk. Children copy specific patterns or designs or draw a hopscotch course.

▽ Use thick sidewalk chalk or egg-shaped pieces of chalk.

Writing and Language: Letter and number writing, spelling

Tripod grasp, planning and organisation (where to start, how big to draw)

Fine Motor Coordination Skills

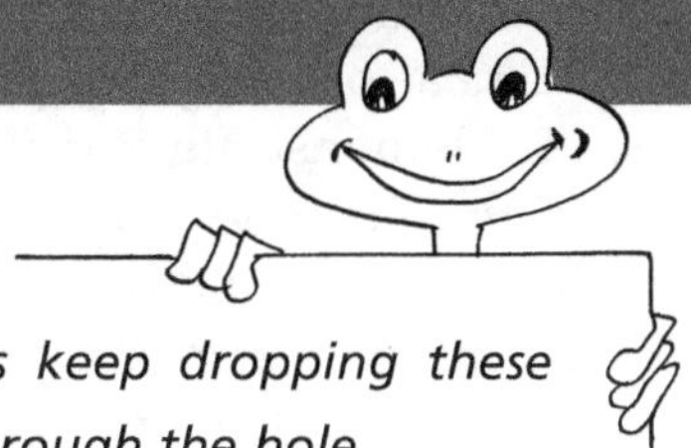

Luke: *Mrs Thompson, my fingers keep dropping these beads and I can't get the string through the hole.*

Luke often has difficulty manipulating small items. Sometimes his hands and fingers move very slowly and awkwardly and it takes much effort for him to complete a fine motor task. Rather than just using his thumb and index finger, he will often use all of his fingers to pick up even small items.

Effective fine motor coordination skills rely on:

- The development of the proper muscles needed to perform the activity.
- A well-developed sensory system ready to perceive the materials being used and provide feedback about the movements being performed.
- The ability to spontaneously plan and sequence movements in order to carry out the task, which is often referred to as fine motor planning.
- The ability to use a functional grasp to successfully complete an activity.
- The ability to process visual information and coordinate it with a motor movement response. This is frequently referred to as eye–hand or visual–motor coordination and integration.
- The ability to manipulate small objects within the hand and with the fingers in a fluent manner, often called speed and manipulation.
- The ability to use the precision side of the hand to hold a pencil and the power side to keep it stable, which we refer to as tripod grasp development.

Children experiencing difficulty with manipulation skills may be observed to have:

- difficulty manipulating objects within the hand
- difficulty stabilising one part of the hand or wrist while simultaneously using the fingers in a fluent manner
- difficulty with isolating finger movements; fingers might appear to 'stick together'
- difficulty maintaining grasp and control of a tool such as a pencil
- difficulty with speed of movement
- difficulty with sequencing movement (Benbow, 1995).

The activities in this section will promote development of skills to specifically enhance fine motor coordination. Because of the nature of these activities there will be overlap with activities in other sections, but the main focus here will be on activities that promote:

- tripod grasp development
- eye–hand coordination
- fine motor speed and manipulation.

TRIPOD GRASP DEVELOPMENT: PENCIL FRIENDS ACTIVITIES

Most of the activities in this section encourage development of a mature tripod grasp, as well as enhance the neat pincer grasp pattern, which involves using the tips of the thumb and index finger. To demonstrate and use the tripod grasp, a child must be able to isolate the 'mover fingers' (thumb, index, and middle fingers) from the 'stabiliser fingers' (ring and pinky fingers). The thumb should oppose the index finger and the middle finger should be just underneath the index finger (see photo on page 78). Encourage children to use their 'pencil friend' (tripod grasp) fingers to perform *all* of these activities, unless otherwise stated. Remember that the ring and pinky fingers should be tucked away from the action.

EYE–HAND COORDINATION: SEE AND DO ACTIVITIES

Combining visual–perceptual and fine motor skills, visual–motor integration and coordination is the ability to synchronise visual information (eyes) with an appropriate motor response (hands) during an activity (Beery, 1997). Of course, when one thinks of eye–hand coordination, most often ball-catching skills or bead threading come to mind. However, children with poor eye–hand coordination may display difficulty with many other fine motor activities requiring visual guidance, such as reproduction of letters and numbers, placement of letters on a line, and cutting accurately along a line. Therefore, when children are performing these activities it is also important to consider their eye movements, such as the ability to maintain their focus on a 'near' task, or change focus from a 'distant' to near task, for example, when copying from a blackboard. These eye movements are called convergence. Difficulty in smoothly visually tracking across the midline from left to right and top to bottom may also significantly impact eye–hand coordination. For some children, weakness in actual visual attention control or a high level of distractability could be contributing factors for poor visual focus. If you feel this to be of significant concern, referral to a paediatrician for further evaluation may be in order.

Note. If you have any doubts about a child's visual–perceptual skills, a thorough examination by an optometrist to check for convergence or visual tracking difficulties is recommended.

FINE MOTOR SPEED AND MANIPULATION: SPEEDY FINGERS ACTIVITIES

Some children may also be observed to have great difficulty in making their fingers move quickly, even when prompted. These children often benefit from activities that incorporate kinaesthetic awareness, such as those found in the Sensory and Planning section, and also from 'timed' games.

Helpful hints

- Outside of this program, most activities can be restructured by setting a specific time limit (for example, 30 seconds), or by giving a set number of objects to be manipulated (such as string 10 beads). Many of the activities in other sections of this manual can also be adapted and used with a timer to increase hand speed and dexterity.
- Fine motor speed and manipulation activities that are timed and even graphed can increase motivation. It is often less stressful for children if they only have to beat their *own* score, and not race against someone else. However, some children have been known to suddenly become very motivated when they have to beat someone else's score, even if it is only the trainers's score. A word of caution though: Some children can become overly anxious when a timing component is introduced. Monitor each child carefully and modify as necessary. The aim of increasing finger speed and manipulation should not be at the expense of a child's feelings of worth or success.

Fine motor coordination activities focus points

When you are working on fine motor coordination activities with children, the following focus points will assist you in observing that the children are performing the activities in the correct manner. These focus points can also be found in card format at the beginning of the Fine Motor Coordination activity cards section, for quick reference. A verbal cue or reminder for you to use is given at the end of each focus point.

- **Bilateral coordination**. Ensure the children are using both sides of their body together, in a smooth, coordinated manner. Ensure that both hands are being used together so that the dominant (worker) hand performs the task and the non-dominant (helper) hand stabilises or assists. **'Two hands'** or **'Where's the helper hand?'**

- **Finger isolation**. Ensure the children can move their fingers independently of each other. **'Just that one finger'** or **'Other fingers away'**

- **Hand dominance**. Take note of which hand each child generally uses. Once established, encourage the children to use their dominant hand to perform the activity, with their non-dominant 'helper' hand either used as a stabiliser or placed behind their back. **'Worker hand only'** or **'Helper hand away'**

- **In-hand manipulation**. Ensure the children are using their thumb and all of their fingers (but not their other hand) to manipulate the object within the palm of their hand. Be aware of children who cannot move objects around within the palm of their hand or bring objects up to their fingertips. **'Fingers only'**

- **Planning and organisation**. Ensure the children have a plan to organise their movement or perform the task. Encourage them to think through the steps. **'What's your plan?'**

- **Pincer grasp**. Ensure the children use the tip of their thumb and index finger. The space between the thumb and fingers should be open and in the shape of an 'O'. **'Pinchy fingers'**

- **Sequencing**. Ensure the children are performing the activity following the correct sequence of movement. **'What comes next?'**

- **Speed**. Ensure the children are able to make their fingers go faster to perform an activity if speed is the focus. **'Speedy fingers'**

- **Thumb flexion**. Ensure the thumb is bent at the middle joint and not overly extended. Explain that you should be able to see the 'mountain on the thumb'. **'Strong thumbs'** or **'Mountain thumb'**

- **Tripod grasp**. Ensure the children use their thumb in opposition with their index and middle fingers. There should be an open space between the thumb and fingers. The ring and little fingers should be tucked away, closer to the palm. The middle finger joints should be bent. **'Pencil fingers'**

- **Visual tracking and focus**. Ensure the children can follow a moving object with just their eyes, without moving their head. Ensure they can keep their visual focus on a task. **'Eyes on the job'**

- **Wrist extension and stability**. Ensure the wrist is not bent in towards the body. It should be slightly extended. **'Wrist up'**

☑ SUPPLIES LIST

For fine motor coordination activities

Items from common supplies box

- ☐ Nuts, dried beans and peas, popcorn kernels
- ☐ Pegs, buttons, beads, small stones
- ☐ Coins, poker chips or counters
- ☐ LEGO®, K'NEX®, Hama beads®
- ☐ Magnetic numbers and letters
- ☐ Paper, tissue paper, card, construction paper
- ☐ Coloured adhesive-backed paper
- ☐ Glue
- ☐ Hole punch
- ☐ Marbles
- ☐ Large tweezers, tongs, chopsticks (joined)
- ☐ String, wool, cotton, yarn
- ☐ Pencils
- ☐ Macaroni, pasta
- ☐ Paperclips
- ☐ Paddlepop sticks, flat toothpicks, coffee stirrers
- ☐ Egg cartons
- ☐ Shape, letter, and number flash cards
- ☐ Sand and containers
- ☐ Scissors
- ☐ Markers
- ☐ Blu Tack (a product of Bostik Australia)
- ☐ Tape

Additional items

- ☐ Zippers, rows of buttons, snappers, and laces, or clothes for dolls or toy animals that have zippers, buttons, snappers, and laces
- ☐ Dolls or toy animals
- ☐ Ello™
- ☐ Macramé string, nylon craft ribbon
- ☐ Barbie® dolls, boys' action figures
- ☐ Locks and keys
- ☐ Spiral stainless steel egg cups or trivets
- ☐ Plastic practice golf balls
- ☐ Wire or chenille sticks (pipe cleaners)
- ☐ Containers with lids
- ☐ Tiddly Winks game (store bought or homemade)
- ☐ Bottles, jars, or containers with narrow mouths
- ☐ Nuts, bolts, and washers (hardware store items), or plastic/wooden toys
- ☐ Miniature marshmallows or gumdrops
- ☐ Pegboard and pegs of different sizes and shapes (commercially available)
- ☐ Pick Up Sticks game (store bought or homemade)
- ☐ Manual pencil sharpener
- ☐ Spinning tops, Doodletop® pens
- ☐ Playing cards and cards from other games
- ☐ Target
- ☐ Shoelace tying board (store bought or home-made) and different-coloured shoelaces
- ☐ Small, coloured stones
- ☐ Straight pins, different types of push pins, pincushions, corkboards

Fine Motor Coordination Activities

CARD 1

Fine Motor Coordination Skills Focus Points

- **Bilateral coordination**. Ensure the children are using both sides of their body together, in a smooth, coordinated manner. Ensure that both hands are being used together so that the dominant (worker) hand performs the task and the non-dominant (helper) hand stabilises or assists. **'Two hands'** or **'Where's the helper hand?'**
- **Finger isolation**. Ensure the children can move their fingers independently of each other. **'Just that one finger'** or **'Other fingers away'**
- **Hand dominance**. Take note of which hand each child generally uses. Once established, encourage the children to use their dominant hand to perform the activity, with their non-dominant 'helper' hand either used as a stabiliser or placed behind their back. **'Worker hand only'** or **'Helper hand away'**

CARD 2

Fine Motor Coordination Skills Focus Points

- **In-hand manipulation.** Ensure the children are using their thumb and all of their fingers (but not their other hand) to manipulate the object within the palm of their hand. Be aware of children who cannot move objects around within the palm of their hand or bring objects up to their fingertips. **'Fingers only'**
- **Planning and organisation**. Ensure the children have a plan to organise their movement or perform the task. Encourage them to think through the steps. **'What's your plan?'**
- **Pincer grasp**. Ensure the children use the tip of their thumb and index finger. The space between the thumb and fingers should be open and in the shape of an 'O'. **'Pinchy fingers'**
- **Sequencing**. Ensure the children are performing the activity following the correct sequence of movement. **'What comes next?'**
- **Speed**. Ensure the children are able to make their fingers go faster to perform an activity if speed is the focus. **'Speedy fingers'**

CARD 3

Fine Motor Coordination Skills Focus Points

- **Thumb flexion**. Ensure the thumb is bent at the middle joint and not overly extended. Explain that you should be able to see the 'mountain on the thumb'. **'Strong thumbs'** or **'Mountain thumb'**
- **Tripod grasp**. Ensure the children use their thumb in opposition with their index and middle fingers. There should be an open space between the thumb and fingers. The ring and little fingers should be tucked away, closer to the palm. The middle finger joints should be bent. **'Pencil fingers'**
- **Visual tracking and focus**. Ensure the children can follow a moving object with just their eyes, without moving their head. Ensure they can keep their visual focus on a task. **'Eyes on the job'**
- **Wrist extension and stability**. Ensure the wrist is not bent in towards the body. It should be slightly extended. **'Wrist up'**

FMC1

Activity 1: Squirrel Game

Tools: Nuts, dried beans, popcorn kernels, small pegs, buttons, coins

Action: With their dominant hand only, children use their fingers to pick up and store small objects such as nuts, beans, small pegs, buttons, and coins in their palm. Remember, only one hand is doing the work.

△ Pick up and store very tiny objects such as grains of uncooked rice.

Mathematics: Counting

In-hand manipulation skills, finger isolation, planning and organisation

FMC2

Activity 2: Button-Up

Tools: Dolls or toy animals with clothes that require buttoning, zipping, snapping, and tying

Action: Have children practise buttoning, snapping, zipping, tying, and other types of fastening by dressing dolls or stuffed toys in clothes. Or, create other fastening games using old clothes with buttons, zippers, studs, and so on.

Hint: Use two different-coloured laces for tying.

△ Decrease the size of the button, and use more complex fasteners.

▽ Use larger buttons. Attach a larger item to the pull tab of a zipper for the children to grip.

Language: Discussion about clothing, how to do a task

Tripod and pincer grasp, bilateral coordination, planning and organisation, sequencing

FMC3

Activity 3: Build It

Tools: LEGO®, K'NEX®, Hama beads®, Ello™

Action: Using the 'building materials' provided, children have to copy a design or, to encourage their imagination skills, create one of their own.

Hint: Use animal or people 'blocks' in the designs to add interest.

△ Create harder and more complex designs; look at a design, remember it, then build it

▽ Create simpler designs; provide step by step modelling

Laterality, Directionality, Language, Mathematics: Top and bottom, right and left, colour recognition, spatial concepts

Tripod grasp, manipulation, bilateral coordination, planning and organisation, visual focus

FMC4

Activity 4: Lock and Key

Tools: Locks and keys

Action: Children fit keys into different locks to open them.

△ Introduce speed: 'How many locks can you undo?'

▽ Provide big keys and big locks. Colour-code locks with keys.

Mathematics: Spatial concepts, size discrimination

Bilateral coordination, lateral pincer grasp (thumb placed to side of the middle joint of the index finger) to hold key, planning and organisation

FMC5

Activity 5: Eggcup Spiral

SEE PHOTO FMC5 ON RESOURCE CD

Tools: Metal spiral eggcups, various-sized beads

Action: Using a pincer grasp, children thread beads onto a metal spiral eggcup. They will enjoy watching the bead spiral its way down the eggcup to the base.

△ For older children who are learning their letters, use alphabet beads. Use this activity to enhance patterning skills, with repetitions of colours, sizes, or numbers of beads.

Mathematics and Writing: Counting beads, patterning, letter identification

Pincer grasp, sequencing, visual tracking, bilateral coordination

FMC6

Activity 6: Knot Funny

Tools: Macramé string, wool, shoelaces, nylon craft ribbon

Action: Children tie a basic knot to make a knot necklace, tie a package, or make craft items, such as a wreath.

△ Have children follow a pattern of knots. Thread beads between knots.

▽ Have children make simple knots on colourful strings.

Science and Mathematics: Sequencing, counting

Grasp and finger strength, sequencing, planning and organisation, bilateral coordination

FMC7

Activity 7: Sorting Stuff

Tools: Beans, beads, coins, magnetic letters and numbers, egg cartons

Action: Using a pincer grasp, children sort different-coloured beans and beads, different coin denominations, different letters, and different numbers into different compartments of an empty egg carton.

△ Give a time frame in which to complete the activity. Place the container on the opposite side of body to their dominant hand to encourage crossing of the midline.

Mathematics and Language: Counting, categorising, object identification.

Pincer grasp, speed, sequencing, bilateral coordination, in-hand manipulation

FMC8

Activity 8: Threaded Golf Balls

Tools: Plastic training golf balls with holes, chenille sticks or thin plastic-coated wire

Action: Thread a 30 cm length of wire through two of the holes on a golf ball, twist it, and tie securely. Using a pincer grasp, children thread the remaining length of the wire in and out of the holes until it is all used up. This is a fantastic and stimulating 3-D threading activity.

Hint: Ensure ends of wire are safely covered.

Laterality and Directionality: Concepts of in/out, left and right, top and bottom

Pincer grasp, eye–hand coordination, visual focus, bilateral coordination, planning and organisation

FMC9

Activity 9: Money in the Bank

Tools: Coins, poker chips, containers with lids, scissors, markers

Action: Using a pincer grasp, children insert coins or poker chips through a slot in a container.

△ Place container on a vertical surface to encourage wrist extension. Make the slot small enough so that the coins or chips fit through it with some resistance. Draw letters or numbers onto poker chips, and have children insert the chips through the slot following a sequence of letters or numbers. Make this a speed challenge: 'How many coins can you get in?'

▽ Increase size of coin or chip and size of slot.

Mathematics and Language: Counting, sorting, letter/number matching

Pincer grasp, bilateral coordination, visual focus, sequencing, hand dominance, speed

FMC10

Activity 10: Tireless Tearing

Tools: Paper

Action: Children use a pincer grasp to tear a piece of paper into strips. These strips can then be used in various ways: (a) scrunch them up with fingertips to make small 'soccer balls' for a finger soccer game in which children have to flick the paper balls into a goal or at a target to score a point, (b) use them for weaving, (c) use them for papier-mâché.

△ Use coarser paper or multiple layers of paper.

▽ Use lightweight paper.

Directionality and Mathematics: Concepts of top to bottom, count the strips

Pincer grasp, bilateral coordination, visual tracking and focus, planning and organisation

FMC11

Activity 11: Load 'Em Up

Tools: Dried peas and beans; popcorn kernels; small, narrow-mouth, screw-top bottles

Action: Children use a pincer grasp to pick up small objects and place them in a bottle through a narrow opening. Also ask the children to unscrew and screw up the lid of the bottle. This is useful for encouraging one hand to act as a stabiliser or helper and the other to act as a mover or worker.

▽ Use a larger container with a wider opening.

Mathematics: Counting

Pincer grasp, bilateral coordination, visual focus, hand dominance, in-hand manipulation

FMC12

Activity 12: Marbles, Tiddly Winks, or Coin Toss Game

Tools: Marbles, coins, Tiddly Winks, targets

Action: Using their thumbs, children flick marbles, Tiddly Winks, or coins on to a target.

Hint: This activity may work better if played on the floor.

△ Make target smaller.

▽ Make target larger.

Mathematics and Language: Count marbles, sorting by colour, colour identification, discuss 'old time' games

Thumb flexion, isolation of movement, wrist stability/extension, hand dominance, visual tracking and focus

FMC13

Activity 13: Archaeology Dig

SEE PHOTO FMC13 ON RESOURCE CD

Tools: Large tweezers or tongs, any small objects (foam or plastic letters, numbers, or shapes; small coloured stones) containers, sand

Action: Children hold tweezers or tongs in a tripod grasp and search for 'buried treasure' in the sand. Helper hand holds the container.

Hint: This activity could also be done in a sandpit during outdoor play, using old kitchen tongs and larger buried objects such as building blocks or stacking cubes.

△ Give a sequence of shapes, letters, numbers, or objects to be found. These can be told to the children before they start as a memory task, or given as a picture on a cue card.

Mathematics and Language: Sorting, counting, object identification

Tripod grasp, bilateral coordination, visual focus, sequencing, hand dominance

FMC14

Activity 14: Jewellery Design

Tools: Beads, macaroni, paper, hole punch, string

Action: String different-shaped and different-sized beads and/or macaroni to make a necklace, or use a hole punch on small pieces of paper that have different letters or numbers drawn on them, and string them to make a word necklace.

Hint: Incorporate this with SH20 activity.

△ Follow a set pattern.

▽ Use larger beads, thicker string/cord/shoelace.

Mathematics and Language: Counting, sorting, letter and number identification

Tripod and pincer grasp on string, bilateral coordination, visual focus, sequencing, in-hand manipulation

FMC15

Activity 15: Wind It Up

Tools: 30 cm pieces of cotton or wool, string, chenille sticks, spools, pencils, Barbie® doll, boys' action figure, Fidget Frog™

Action: Children use a pincer grasp and wind cotton, string, or wool onto a spool or pencil so that it is covered, or bandage up a doll's limb.

△ Wind around ridges of a bolt for more precision.

Mathematics and Language: Measure length of string when stretched out before wrapping as compared to length of string when wrapped, discussion about caring for the injured and health workers

Pincer grasp on string, bilateral coordination, visual focus

FMC16

Activity 16: Construction Capers

Tools: Nuts, bolts, washers

Action: Using a tripod grasp, children assemble an assortment of nuts and bolts.

△ Use only thumb and index fingers to manipulate the nuts and bolts. Introduce speed: 'How many can you put together before the music plays?'

▽ Use larger nuts and bolts.

Mathematics: Counting and sorting

Tripod and pincer grasp, bilateral coordination, visual focus, sequencing, in-hand manipulation, hand dominance

FMC17

Activity 17: Paperclip Link Up

Tools: Paperclips, coloured adhesive-backed paper (optional)

Action: Depending on the size of the paperclips, children use a tripod or pincer grasp to link the paperclips together to make all sorts of chains, connectors, or jewellery.

△ Cut up small strips of coloured adhesive-backed paper (a great cutting activity) and, once linked, cover each paper clip with it to make coloured jewellery, chains, or connectors. Reproduce a coloured pattern from a model or from memory.

Mathematics: Count strung-together clips or chains (it may be fun to gather statistics and chart progress)

Tripod or pincer grasp, sequencing, bilateral coordination, visual focus

FMC18

Activity 18: Molecular Builder

Tools: Flat toothpicks; coffee stirrers; gumdrops, miniature marshmallows, or Blu Tack (a product of Bostik Australia)

Action: Create models with flat toothpicks or coffee stirrers connected with miniature marshmallows, gumdrops, or Blu Tack (a product of Bostik Australia).

△ Copy a design.

Mathematics and Language: Count number of toothpicks or stirrers used, spatial relations, geometry, sorting gumdrops by colour, colour identification

Pincer grasp, bilateral coordination, visual focus, sequencing, in-hand manipulation, hand dominance

FMC19

Activity 19: Peg Board Play

Tools: Pegs, pegboards

Action: Children use a tripod or pincer grasp to insert different-sized and different-shaped pegs into a pegboard.

△ Reproduce a sequence or pattern. Have children remember a pattern and then reproduce it. Have children create and follow their own patterns. Place pegboard vertically to encourage wrist extension.

Mathematics: Pattern replication and design, shape identification, spatial concepts

Tripod grasp, bilateral coordination to stabilise pegboard, hand dominance, in-hand manipulation

FMC20

Activity 20: Pick Up Sticks Game

Tools: Pick Up Sticks game

Action: Using a pincer grasp to pick up the sticks, children play the game. (Pick Up Sticks is a commercially available game in which players aim to pick up one stick at a time from a pile of sticks without moving any of the other sticks.)

Mathematics and Language: Spatial relations, colour identification

Pincer grasp, planning and organisation, hand dominance, bilateral coordination, visual focus

FMC21

Activity 21: Pencil Sharpening

Tools: Blunt pencils, manual pencil sharpener

Action: Give children a handful of blunt pencils to sharpen. This is actually trickier than it seems for children, as it requires great coordination between the two hands, one acts as a stabiliser and the other as the worker, and checking when the pencil is sharp and stopping.

Hint: Give direct guidelines, such as 'Three turns of the pencil, stop and check if it is sharp. If yes, stop and get a new pencil, if no, do three more turns. Ask children to bring their own pencil cases to the session.

Mathematics: How many pencils can be sharpened in a session?

Tripod grasp, bilateral coordination, planning and organisation

FMC22

Activity 22: Top It Off

Tools: Tops, Doodletop® pens, paper

Action: Have children practise spinning a top or Doodletop® pen with their index finger, middle finger, and thumb.

△ If using a Doodletop® pen, cover the desk with paper and ask children to spin the pen to cover all of the paper, not just the spot directly in front of them, with squiggles.

Language: Colour identification, design description

Tripod grasp, planning and organisation, hand dominance, in-hand manipulation, visual tracking and focus

FMC23

Activity 23: Card Shark

Tools: Playing cards, cards from other games

Action: Depending on the cards being used, children shuffle, deal, or sort cards into various categories.

△ Introduce speed: 'How many cards can you deal or sort in X number of seconds?'. Increase the amount of categories

▽ Use stiffer cards.

Mathematics and Language: Count shuffling or sorting repetitions (it may be fun to gather statistics and chart progress), sorting, classifying

Bilateral coordination, speed, pincer or tripod grasp to pick up individual cards, sequencing

FMC24

Activity 24: Tissue Paper Art

Tools: Tissue paper, construction paper, glue

Action: Children wad up small pieces of coloured tissue paper with their fingers and then glue them onto a larger sheet of paper to make a 3-D picture or fill in a colouring picture or geometric shape.

Hint: Use paper strips torn in a previous session.

△ Use only a pincer grasp. Attach the background paper to a vertical surface to build shoulder strength while doing this activity.

Mathematics, Language, Art: Counting, colour identification, creative expression

Pincer grasp, wrist extension, hand dominance, planning and organisation

FMC25

Activity 25: Wonderful Weaving

Tools: Yarn, string, paper, chenille sticks, commercially available plastic baskets with a pattern of holes in them.

Action: Use paper, string, yarn, or chenille sticks to create lovely projects by weaving in and out or over and under the holes in the basket. Encourage children to verbalise the steps, such as 'over and under', to help with planning.

Hint: This can also be a group project by having each child continue on from the last child.

△ Have children follow a pattern of colours to be threaded.

Language and Mathematics: Spatial concepts, patterning

Tripod grasp, planning and organisation, sequencing, bilateral coordination, visual tracking and focus

FMC26

Activity 26: Shoelace Tying

Tools: Shoelace tying board (a sturdy cardboard square with two holes for the laces to go through), two different-coloured shoelaces

Action: Stabilise the board and teach children how to tie the laces, step by step. Specific instruction on method varies, so use trial and error to see which one works for each child: (a) bunny ears (make two loops first) or (b) single loop and wrap around. Make sure the children initially make a smaller loop and leave a 'longer tail' (the end of the lace), so that wrapping around becomes easier. Pull both loops at the end to even up loops and tails.

Hint: Try a backward or forward chaining method to teach this skill (refer to Sensory and Planning Skills section).

Laterality and Language: Right and left, verbal sequencing

Neat or lateral pincer grasp, planning and organisation, sequencing, bilateral coordination, thumb flexion

FMC27

Activity 27: Pin Designs

Tools: Straight pins, different types of push pins, plastic golf tees; pincushions, corkboards, or polystyrene foam packaging; shape, letter, or number flash cards

Action: Children pick up pins from in a container using a neat pincer grasp, then copy patterns by pushing pins into a pincushion/corkboard.

Hint: This activity may require close supervision. Plastic golf tees may be used as a substitute.

△ Colour-code the patterns, such as using all red-tipped pins.

▽ Draw shapes on a piece of paper and place on top of the corkboard or polystyrene foam as a guide for where to push in the pins.

Mathematics and Language: Spatial relations, pattern copying, colour identification

Pincer grasp, planning and organisation, sequencing, bilateral coordination

Pencil to Paper Skills

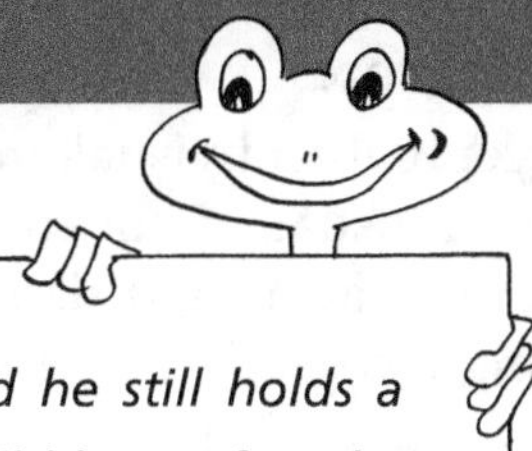

Parent: *Lance is five years old now and he still holds a crayon with his whole hand and just scribbles. In fact, he really is very resistant to any drawing activities. Is this just a 'boy thing'?*

Lance is typical of many children (often, but not always, boys) showing little or no interest in drawing tasks. There can be a number of reasons for this. He has obviously not yet developed a refined dynamic tripod grasp for holding writing tools, which means that he will have reduced control and ability to draw small details. Because he has no interest in this activity, it also means that he has had fewer chances to develop appropriate skills.

For children of this age there are a number of factors that need to be considered as they develop writing skills. These include:

- Their level of interest and motivation in drawing and writing.
- Their hand dominance. Although it is not always firmly established at this age, the majority of children will be showing a strong tendency towards using a certain hand by the age of three years.
- Their ability to hold different writing tools/implements, such as crayons and pencils, using a tripod grasp.
- Their visual–motor skills or ability to perceive a shape or letter visually and then reproduce it by using a motor response, as in copying or drawing from memory.
- Their ability to visually focus on the page, with both eyes working together.
- Their ability to concentrate.
- Their ability to use one hand as a stabilising 'helper' hand to hold the paper still and the other 'worker' hand to move the pencil.

The act of handwriting requires the complex integration of many skills and it is not within the scope of this manual to go into great detail regarding this. However, children displaying handwriting difficulties may do so for a number of reasons (Benbow, 1995; Cornhill & Case-Smith, 1996; Feder, Majnemer, & Synnes, 2000; Hammerschmidt & Sudsawald, 2004; Marr & Dimeo, 2006; McGarrigle, 2006). These may include the following:

- poor sitting position
- reduced attention control

- sensory deficits such as poor finger awareness affecting joint position sense and movement sense
- specific visual deficits such as reduced visual acuity, poor visual tracking, and/or visual convergence
- visual–perceptual and visual–motor difficulties such as weakness in memory for motor patterns, poor visual–motor coordination, weakness in visual–spatial awareness affecting even spacing and sizing of letters and words, and reduced visual discrimination affecting recognition of letters and differences between similar looking letters such as 'b' and 'd', 'p' and 'q'
- poor shoulder and wrist stability
- poor pencil control due to low muscle tone and strength in the hands
- inefficient pencil grasp.

Following are some concrete suggestions and guidelines to help improve some of the problem areas listed above.

POSITIONING, POSITIONING, POSITIONING!

- Encourage children to be aware of good sitting posture or cue children to check their posture before commencing writing or drawing tasks (refer to Section A of this manual). Be sure to double-check their feet position.
- Ensure non-writing 'helper' hand is stabilising the paper.
- Paper should be tilted slightly so that it is in line or parallel with the writing arm.
- Head should be in the midline. If a child's head is excessively tilted to one side during writing tasks, referral to an optometrist to examine visual convergence is recommended.

USING A TRIPOD GRASP: PENCIL FRIENDS

A brief glance around the classroom will indicate that many children do not hold their pencils with a mature, dynamic tripod grasp (see photo below). The dynamic tripod grasp is generally considered to be the most efficient grasp for children aged five years or older, although some other modified grasps may be acceptable if they do not interfere with function and fluency.

Features of the Dynamic Tripod Grasp

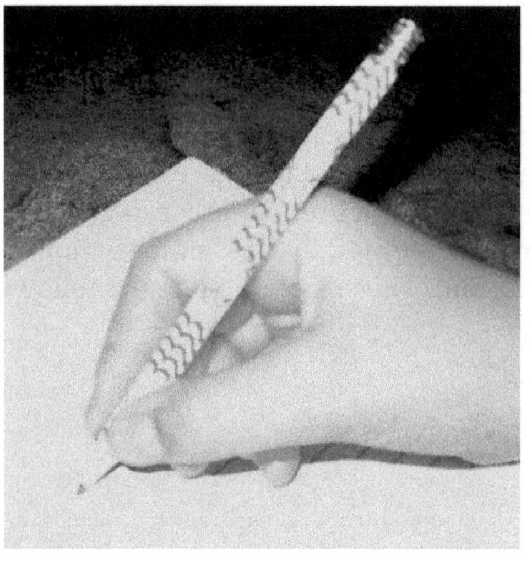

- The pencil should be held lightly in a triangle position with the index finger on the top (driver's seat), thumb meeting the tip of the index finger (passenger seat), and middle finger supporting the pencil underneath (backseat).
- The fingers should be approximately 25 mm from the point. Tape can be placed around the pencil or a soft cylindrical comfort grip can be used to help with correct finger placement.

Helpful hint

- One of the essentials of any functional pencil grasp is to maintain an open web space (the area between the thumb and index finger). If the web space is closed there will be limited movement initiated from the distal (end) finger joints and pencil control and smooth writing movements will be compromised. Some modified grasps, which are non-traditional, may still be functional if the web space remains open.

- The shaft of the pencil should rest on the side of the index finger just near the large knuckle, not in the web space between the thumb and index finger.
- Writing movement should come primarily from the middle and distal fingertip joints, *not* from the wrist. The forearm and wrist should be supported on the desk and in a neutral or slightly extended position, bent away from the body and definitely *not* flexed or bent towards the body.

Helpful hint

- To promote improved wrist position for children whose wrist is very flexed or bent, a slope board or large ringbinder can be used. Cover this in funky paper. A small sticker can also be placed on the outer edge of the wrist as a cue for children that it is to remain on the desktop.
- Commercially available pencil grips may be useful for promoting a better grasp. However, with consultation from an occupational therapist, for long-term benefit it is wise to look at underlying reasons for poor pencil grip, such as reduced hand strength or lowered muscle tone, and work on these as well.
- For younger children, it may be beneficial to introduce thicker drawing tools before narrow ones. Triangular crayons, colouring pencils, sidewalk chalk, chunky pencils, novelty pencils, and magic markers are a great way to encourage drawing. As skills develop, introduce narrower tools to help refine the tripod grasp.

LETTER AND NUMBER FORMATION: WRITING RIGHT

As letter formation and teaching methods vary throughout the world, please refer to the specific writing programs used by your state or school district. When choosing activities for this section, it would be most beneficial to use the letter, number, sight, or spelling words that are currently being used in your classroom.

Remember that there are a number of sensory writing tasks in the Sensory and Planning Activities section that can also be used to reinforce shape, letter, and number formation.

The following activities and tips are useful ways for children to initially learn to write letters and numbers and to encourage them to write between the lines:

- Reinforce letter shape by using letter stories, such as '"m" is for mountain, top to bottom, up and over the mountain, up and over the mountain'.
- Use a visual picture to accompany the letter so that there is another memory trigger.

- Reinforce the motor pattern for forming letters and numbers by having children trace over clay or sandpaper letters or numbers with their fingers, drawing in the air, and writing letters with their eyes closed. Be sure to highlight the fact that all of the letters except for 'e' start at the top.
- When transitioning from writing letters on unlined paper to lined paper, try these ideas:
  - Create a strong visual contrast by colouring the area between the lines in different colours. Use a colouring pencil to colour in blue between the blue lines and red for the top and bottom line areas. This gives children defined areas for their letters to begin and finish in. It also encourages them to be aware of when they go out of the correct writing area on the paper.
  - Give points when the children 'hit' the line at the right place. If you make this into a pinball game, the children love to add up their hit points. An accompanying 'ping' sound by the trainer can also be fun and motivating.
  - Use a unique, Australian-designed, Writing Line Cat Stamp to show line placement and identify head, body, and tail letters. This stamp can be made for different types of lines and has been a great success. For further information visit www.fingergym.resources.com
  - Above all, it is most important that children see writing as an expression of their ideas and not just focus on the mechanics of writing. For children who continue to have major difficulties with the writing process as they proceed through higher grades, alternative forms of communication may be considered. An occupational therapy assessment would be beneficial at this point.

Pencil to paper activities focus points

When you are working on pencil to paper activities with children, the following focus points will assist you in observing that the children are using the correct muscles and performing the activities in the correct manner. These focus points can also be found in card format at the beginning of the Pencil to Paper activity cards section, for quick reference. A verbal cue or reminder for you to use is given at the end of each focus point.

- **Bilateral coordination**. Ensure the children are using both hands. The worker or dominant hand should be holding the pencil and the helper or non-dominant hand should be stabilising the paper. **'Two hands'**
- **Crossing midline when writing**. Ensure the children can write smoothly from left to right across the page by sliding their forearm without moving their whole body, or excessively tilting their head. **'Left to right across the page'** or **'Body still, cross over'**
- **Hand dominance**. Take note of which hand is generally used to hold the pencil. Encourage skill development by encouraging the children to use their other (helper) hand to stabilise the paper. **'Use your pencil hand'**
- **Letter starting points**. Ensure the children begin their letters or numbers at the correct point. **'Where does it start?'**
- **Memory strategy**. Encourage the children to remember what letters look like by describing them, associating them with a letter picture, or drawing them in the air. **'Close your eyes and see the letter in your head'**
- **Paper stabilisation**. Ensure the helper hand is holding the paper steady on the desk. **'Paper steady'** or **'Helper hand on the paper'**
- **Pencil control**. Ensure the children are using smooth, controlled movements to guide the pencil. Take note of speed, visual focus, pencil grasp, and wrist support. **'Smooth and steady writing'**
- **Posture**. Ensure the children are sitting with their body and head in the midline, arms supported on the desk, and eyes approximately at elbow distance from the page. **'Sitting tall and straight'**
- **Tripod grasp**. Ensure the children use their thumb in opposition with their index and middle fingers. There should be an open space (called the web space) between the thumb and fingers. The ring and little fingers should be tucked away, closer to the palm. The middle finger joints should be bent. **'Pencil fingers'**
- **Visual focus**. Ensure the children keep their visual focus on the writing task. Take note of any unusual head positioning to one side during writing tasks. **'Eyes on the job'.**
- **Wrist position**. Ensure the wrist is supported on the desk in slight extension and not bent towards the body or held up in the air. **'Wrist on the desk'**
- **Planning and organisation**. This focus point will vary according to the specific activity. Verbal cues might include **'Does everything fit?'** or **'How can you start this job?'.**
- **Self-monitoring**. Encourage the children to look over their work and appraise it. **'How do you think you've done?'** or **'Have you checked your job?'**

SUPPLIES LIST

For pencil to paper activities

Items from common supplies box

- ☐ Paper, card
- ☐ Crayons, markers, pens, coloured pencils, lead pencils
- ☐ Paint
- ☐ Pencil grips
- ☐ Crayola Colour Changeables® (marker pens)
- ☐ Overwriters®
- ☐ String, wool
- ☐ Whiteboard, whiteboard pens
- ☐ Chalkboard, chalk, and eraser
- ☐ Magnetic numbers, letters, and pictures
- ☐ Blu Tack (a product of Bostik Australia)
- ☐ Magna Doodle®
- ☐ Perspex® or clear plastic folders
- ☐ Stamping pens

Additional items

- ☐ Shape templates (see resource CD)
- ☐ Hand template (see resource CD)
- ☐ Wooden craft shape templates
- ☐ Leaves, ferns
- ☐ Scribble pattern sheets
- ☐ Pre-drawn patterns (store bought and copied or homemade)
- ☐ Newspaper or magazine text
- ☐ Symmetrical drawing reproducible pages
- ☐ Tracing paper, carbon paper
- ☐ Fidget the Frog™ template (see resource CD)
- ☐ Stickers
- ☐ Maze templates (see resource CD or homemade)
- ☐ Tessellating (geometric) pattern colouring sheets (store bought or homemade)
- ☐ Colouring-in pictures
- ☐ Find the Hidden Objects pictures (commecially availables)
- ☐ Pre-writing or writing worksheets
- ☐ Small whiteboards/ blackboard
- ☐ Magnetic drawing boards
- ☐ Blindfold

Pencil to Paper Activities

CARD 1

Pencil to Paper Skills Focus Points

- **Bilateral coordination**. Ensure the children are using both hands. The worker or dominant hand should be holding the pencil and the helper or non-dominant hand should be stabilising the paper. **'Two hands'**
- **Crossing midline when writing**. Ensure the children can write smoothly from left to right across the page by sliding their forearm without moving their whole body or excessively tilting their head. **'Left to right across the page'** or **'Body still, cross over'**
- **Hand dominance**. Take note of which hand is generally used to hold the pencil. Encourage skill development by encouraging the children to use their other (helper) hand to stabilise the paper. **'Use your pencil hand'**
- **Letter starting points.** Ensure the children begin their letters or numbers at the correct point. **'Where does it start?'**

CARD 2

Pencil to Paper Skills Focus Points

- **Memory strategy**. Encourage the children to remember what letters look like by describing them, associating them with a letter picture, or drawing them in the air. **'Close your eyes and see the letter in your head'**
- **Paper stabilisation**. Ensure the helper hand is holding the paper steady on the desk. **'Paper steady'** or **'Helper hand on the paper'**
- **Pencil control**. Ensure the children are using smooth, controlled movements to guide the pencil. Take note of speed, visual focus, pencil grasp, and wrist support. **'Smooth and steady writing'**
- **Posture**. Ensure the children are sitting with their body and head in the midline, arms supported on the desk, and eyes approximately at elbow distance from the page. **'Sitting tall and straight'**

CARD 3

Pencil to Paper Skills Focus Points

- **Tripod grasp**. Ensure the children use their thumb in opposition with their index and middle fingers. There should be an open space (called the web space) between the thumb and fingers. The ring and little fingers should be tucked away, closer to the palm. The middle finger joints should be bent. **'Pencil fingers'**
- **Visual focus**. Ensure the children keep their visual focus on the writing task. Take note of any unusual head positioning to one side during writing tasks. **'Eyes on the job'**
- **Wrist position**. Ensure the wrist is supported on the desk in slight extension and not bent towards the body or held up in the air. **'Wrist on the desk'**
- **Planning and organisation**. This focus point will vary according to the specific activity. Verbal cues might include **'Does everything fit?'** or **'How can you start this job?'**.
- **Self-monitoring.** Encourage the children to look over their work and appraise it. **'How do you think you've done?'** or **'Have you checked your job?'**

PP1

Activity 1: Trace and Colour Designs

SEE PHOTO PP1 ON RESOURCE CD

Tools: Paper, wooden craft shape templates, crayons, markers

Action: Children colour in different shapes that they have traced around. Encourage children to plan where they will place the template on the paper. This activity could be done over two sessions.

△ Use a shape and corresponding colour grid for matching.

▽ Colour shapes by number or letter.

Language and Mathematics: Letter and number recognition, count shapes coloured in

Hand dominance, tripod grasp, paper stabilisation, pencil control, wrist position, planning and organisation, crossing midline when writing, posture, bilateral coordination

PP2

Activity 2: Leaf Designs

Tools: Leaves, ferns, paper, crayons, pencils, paint

Action: Collect a variety of leaves or ferns and (a) trace around a leaf and colour in the outline, (b) place a leaf under paper and rub crayon over the top, (c) paint a leaf and then 'print' it on to a clean sheet of paper, (d) copy a leaf; use the leaf as a model. Then, children compare their leaf design to the original.

Science, Language, Mathematics: Nature and seasons, comparing and contrasting, counting

Hand dominance, tripod grasp, paper stabilisation, pencil control, wrist position, planning and organisation, crossing midline when writing, posture, bilateral coordination

PP3

Activity 3: Rainbow Race Track

Tools: SP17 (lazy eight) or PP18 templates (see resource CD), coloured pencils, crayons, Crayola Colour Changeables® (marker pens)

Action: Children draw between 'roads' multiple times using different-coloured pencils, crayons, or Changeables® marker pens.

△ Decrease width of the path and use more complex curves and angles

▽ Widen the path and use fewer curves

Laterality and Directionality: Turning in different directions to navigate the road.

Hand dominance, tripod grasp, paper stabilisation, pencil control, wrist position, crossing midline when writing, posture

PP4

Activity 4: Show Your Hand

Tools: Pencils, markers, paper, cardboard, string/wool, hand template

Action: Children trace around their own hands or around a hand template.

Hint: Children can take this hand pattern with them to the 'cutting station' to be used for the cutting activity.

△ Draw finger people/families on each of the different fingers. Trace onto cardboard, cut out hand shape, and paste on string or wool for hair or decoration.

Mathematics and Language: Counting fingers, talk about families

Hand dominance, tripod grasp, paper stabilisation, pencil control, wrist position, crossing midline when writing, posture, planning and organisation, bilateral coordination

PP5

Activity 5: Scribble Pictures

SEE PHOTO PP5 ON RESOURCE CD

Tools: Black crayons/markers/pencils, coloured markers/pencils, paper

Action: Children (or trainer) draw a scribble-like overlapping pattern on a piece of paper. Children then trace over the outline with a black coloured pencil or crayon and colour in the different sections in a variety of colours.

△ Overlap the lines so that sections are smaller. Use a shape, letter, or number grid for children to follow as they colour in different sections.

▽ Have larger, less intricate sections to colour.

Language and Mathematics: Letter, word, shape, and number concepts

Hand dominance, sustaining a tripod grasp, paper stabilisation, pencil control, wrist position, crossing midline when writing, posture

PP6

Activity 6: Whiteboard Designs

Tools: Metal-based whiteboard; magnetic letters, numbers, and pictures; whiteboard pens

Action: Place magnetic pictures, letters, and numbers on a metal-based whiteboard. Children draw a line from one picture to the next. To encourage improved wrist extension and stability, the board can be hung vertically on a wall or door.

△ Circle all of the even numbers, join up the letters in alphabetical order, or sequentially connect numbers by 1s or 2s.

Language and Writing: Letter, number, and picture recognition

Hand dominance, tripod grasp, pencil control, wrist position, crossing midline when writing, posture, visual focus

PP7

Activity 7: Let's Magna Doodle® Pictures

SEE PHOTO PP7 ON RESOURCE CD

Tools: Pre-drawn patterns/templates, Magna Doodle®, paper

Action: Draw some patterns on a strip of paper (or use template on resource CD) and stick them down the left side of the Magna Doodle® or at the top. Children continue patterns using the Magna Doodle® pen.

Hint: This activity is great for kids with poor pencil control who get easily frustrated — they can just erase and begin again.

△ Position Magna Doodle® vertically to encourage wrist extension.

▽ Draw a line between two dots from top to bottom, left to right.

Writing and Language: Left to right, top to bottom concepts

Hand dominance, tripod grasp, wrist position, crossing midline when writing, visual focus, posture

PP8

Activity 8: Letter/Number Circle

Tools: Random letters typed on a sheet of paper (or use templates on resource CD), newspaper clippings, magazine articles, clear plastic folder or sheet of perspex®.

Action: Children circle designated letters on a page of random letters or in a paragraph from a newspaper or magazine article. For example, 'Just circle all the "b's" in red'.

△ Try having a combination of commonly confused letters such as 'b' and 'd', 'p' and 'q'. Circle each letter with a different colour.

Writing and Mathematics: Letter recognition, count letter combinations

Hand dominance, tripod grasp, paper stabilisation, pencil control, wrist position, crossing midline when writing, planning and organisation (such as scanning from left to right), posture

PP9

Activity 9: Tessellating Patterns

Tools: Commercially available tessellating (geometric) pattern colouring sheets or homemade pattern sheets, colouring pencils

Action: Children use different colours to produce patterns.

△ Use a shape, letter, number, or sight words grid for children to follow as they colour in different sections.

▽ Provide simpler designs.

Language, Mathematics, Art: Letter, word, shape, and number recognition/matching concepts; spatial concepts

Hand dominance, sustaining a tripod grasp, pencil control, wrist position, paper stabilisation, posture

PP10

Activity 10: Hot and Cold Pictures

Tools: White paper, crayons, markers

Action: Fold a piece of white paper in half. Designate one side Hot and one side Cold. Draw the same picture, such as a house, on both sides. Children colour in the 'hot' picture using hot colours like red, yellow, orange, brown, hot pink, and black and the 'cold' picture using cold colours like light blue, green, purple, white, and pastel pink.

Language and Art: Compare and contrast, colours

Hand dominance, sustaining a tripod grasp, pencil control, wrist position, paper stabilisation, planning and organisation, posture, bilateral coordination

PP11

Activity 11: Symmetrical Drawing

Tools: Paper, crayons, markers

Action: Fold a piece of paper in half. Draw half a picture on one side of the fold. Children complete the other half of the picture.

Hint: A Magna Doodle® could also be used in this activity.

△ Increase the complexity and details of the picture, for example, a person.

Mathematics: Symmetry

Hand dominance, tripod grasp, pencil control, paper stabilisation, wrist position, planning and organisation, posture, bilateral coordination

PP12

Activity 12: See-Through Writing

SEE PHOTO PP12 ON RESOURCE CD

Tools: Paper, pens, clear plastic folders, perspex®, whiteboard marker, pre-drawn or commercial mazes, classroom letter/number worksheets

Action: Draw a shape, letter, number, or word design on paper or use classroom worksheets. Place templates between sheets of a clear plastic folder or under a piece of perspex®. Children trace over design with a whiteboard marker.

△ Increase complexity of designs and patterns.

Writing, Language, Laterality, Directionality: Reinforce shape, letter, and number identification and up and down and left and right concepts.

Hand dominance, tripod grasp, pencil control, paper stabilisation, wrist position, planning and organisation, posture

PP13

Activity 13: Carbon Copy Trace Over

Tools: Tracing paper, carbon paper, pens

Action: Using tracing paper on top and carbon paper underneath, children trace over a picture to make a 'photocopy'. Children quickly learn the importance of their helper hand in this activity.

▽ Secure the picture underneath.

Laterality and Directionality: Up/down, left/right concepts

Hand dominance, tripod grasp, pencil control, wrist position, paper stabilisation, crossing midline when writing, planning and organisation, posture

PP14

Activity 14: Trace Around Fidget™

Tools: Fidget the Frog™ template, paper, pencils

Action: Place template on the paper and children trace around Fidget™ with their pencil. Encourage them to hold the template with their helper hand.

▽ Use Blue Tack (a product of Bostik Australia) or tape to stabilise the template.

Writing and Language: Use Fidget™ to stimulate discussion on amphibians.

Hand dominance, tripod grasp, pencil control, wrist position, paper stabilisation, crossing midline when writing, planning and organisation, bilateral coordination

PP15

Activity 15: Copy That!

Tools: Small whiteboards or blackboards, magnetic drawing boards, paper, pencils

Action: Children copy words, short sentences, or other simple patterns from a small whiteboard or blackboard mounted vertically in front of them. Encourage children to compare their work with the original model.

△ Cover up the design after 10 seconds for children to draw from memory.

Language, Writing, Memory: Reinforce copying skills, verbal rehearsal and memory strategies

Hand dominance, tripod grasp, pencil control, wrist position, visual focus, memory strategy, paper stabilisation, planning and organisation, self-monitoring

PP16

Activity 16: Letter Connectors

Tools: Colourful stickers/stamping pens, paper, pens, markers

Action: Place stickers or stamp shapes at strategic points on the paper and have children connect them with lines to create shapes, letters, and numbers. (The children could prepare the stamping sheets beforehand as another activity.)

Hint: Sheets could also be placed under perspex® or clear plastic sheets so they can be reused.

Writing, Mathematics, Language: Letter, number, and word formation

Hand dominance, tripod grasp, paper stabilisation, pencil control, wrist position, crossing midline when writing, planning and organisation, posture

PP17

Activity 17: Overwriter® Pens and Crayons

Tools: Crayola Colour Changeables® (marker pens) or Overwriters®, paper

Action: Write letters, numbers, or words with one colour and have children trace over them with the Changeables® or Overwriters® markers.

Writing and Language: Letter and word formation, written expression

Hand dominance, tripod grasp, pencil control, wrist position, correct starting points of letters/numbers, paper stabilisation

PP18

Activity 18: Crazy Mazes

Tools: Template mazes (see resource CD or homemade), pencils, markers, stickers

Action: Children have to plan the way as they draw through the maze.

△ Choose mazes with complex curves and angles. Draw coloured spots, shapes, letters, numbers, or sight words along the maze. Children have to circle (or place a sticker on) a specified item as they go through the maze. Children score a point for each correct answer.

▽ Use or make simple mazes that follow a straight line, corners, or curves.

Language and Mathematics: Letter and number recognition

Hand dominance, tripod grasp, pencil control, wrist position, planning and organisation, paper stabilisation, crossing midline when writing, visual focus

PP19

Activity 19: Hidden Picture Games

Tools: Find the Hidden Objects pictures, pencils, stamping pens

Action: Find and circle specified objects with a pencil or stamping pen.

△ Choose harder to find, more obscure hidden objects pictures.

▽ Choose simpler and more obvious hidden objects pictures.

Language: Object identification and naming

Hand dominance, tripod grasp, pencil control, wrist position, planning and organisation, paper stabilisation, visual focus

PP20

Activity 20: Mystery Writer Game

Tools: Chalkboard, chalk, blindfold

Action: Children are blindfolded* and stand at the chalkboard while the trainer guides their hand to write a letter or number on the board. The aim is for the children to guess the letter/number they have written, just by the movement.

▽ Provide letter formation hints while writing or provide sounds.

Writing, Language, Memory: Letter/number formation

Hand dominance, tripod grasp, wrist position, starting points of letters and numbers,

*Do not use blindfold if a child objects to it. Ask them to close their eyes.

PP21

Activity 21: Shadow Writing

Tools: Chalkboard, different-coloured chalk, eraser

Action: Draw shapes, letters, numbers, or words on a chalkboard and then lightly erase them so just a light outline is visible. Have children draw over the erased shapes, letters, numbers, or words several times in different-coloured chalk.

Writing, Mathematics, Language: Letter, number, and word formation

Hand dominance, tripod grasp, pencil control, wrist position, starting points of letters and numbers, visual focus

Cutting Skills

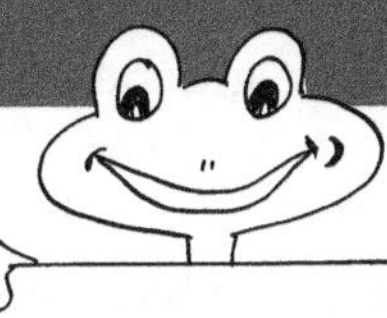

Teacher: *Taylor, remember that the worker hand needs to go 'thumb up to the sky' when you cut with scissors.*

Taylor always turns her cutting hand down so that her thumb points to the ground when she cuts. Not only does this position make it hard for Taylor to cut neatly and precisely, it is uncomfortable and stressful to the joints in her hand and forearm.

Children may have difficulty with cutting for a number of reasons. These include:

- difficulty using the two sides of the hand simultaneously, that is, the thumb and middle finger opening the blades in single loop scissors, with the index finger stabilising under the bottom blade and the other fingers acting as stabilisers
- poor bilateral coordination, that is, using two sides of the body in a coordinated manner so that one hand stabilises and manipulates the paper and the other hand manipulates the scissors
- poor motor planning and visual–motor coordination
- poor hand strength
- poor wrist stability, that is, wrist is bent towards the body (Benbow, 1995)
- reduced attention/visual focus
- using scissors that are an inappropriate size or weight; this can include scissors that have blades that are too long.

Note. As there is an abundance of commercially available resources, this section will not give a large number of specific cutting activities, but rather some guidelines and suggestions to enhance scissors skills.

Before commencing cutting activities, it is important to look at how the child is holding the scissors:

Note. The following suggestions are based on single loop scissors.

- The thumb and middle finger should be placed into the loops only as far as the end knuckles. A visual cue such as tape or a mark can be used. (In scissors with a double loop at the bottom and a single loop at the top, both the index and middle fingers should be placed in the bottom loop.)
- The index finger should be held under the bottom handle to support the scissors and assist in closing them. (This is not applicable in scissors with a double loop at the bottom.)
- The wrist should be slightly *extended*, not bent towards the body.
- The forearm should be on its side; the palm should *not* be facing down.

- Remember the 'thumbs up' position (both the thumb in the scissor loop and the thumb holding the paper) when using scissors.
- It is also necessary to look at how the non-dominant hand is holding the paper. The paper should be grasped between the thumb and index finger, with the thumb on top.

Helpful hint

- Some children have great difficulty knowing when to move their helper hand up the paper as they cut so that the paper remains stable. Starting with straight line cutting, draw short lines at even distances (about 5 cm apart) all the way up the edge of the page. When the scissors reach a line marker, the helper hand must also move up the page.

THE PROGRESSION OF CUTTING SKILLS

- Placing scissors correctly on hands
- Opening and closing the scissors
- Snipping along the edge of a piece of paper
- Cutting across a piece of paper (forward motion)
- Cutting between two lines
- Cutting along a thick and a thin line
- Cutting around corners
- Cutting simple geometric shapes such as a square or triangle
- Cutting gentle curves
- Cutting around a circle, beginning with large circles and progressing to small circles
- Cutting increasingly complex combinations of shapes and angles

Once a child masters snipping and straight cutting across a piece of paper, it is time to introduce cutting around corners and curves. This is often the point when children with poor visual–motor coordination and planning difficulties demonstrate difficulty with scissors tasks. It may appear as if they do not seem to know which way to turn the paper and finish up a cutting activity with their body in a knot. The following may help.

HINTS: A FEW SCISSORS SNIPPETS

- Have the child practise actually placing their fingers correctly in the scissors.
- Have the child practise opening and closing the scissors before introducing paper.
- To encourage the correct wrist and hand position, use a verbal cue such as 'thumbs up' or 'wrist up'. Initially you might have to provide physical assistance to show the child the correct position and help them keep this position during the cutting process.
- For initial training or for children who cannot manage coordinating both hands, it may also be helpful for the child to position the scissors on the desk like dressmaker's scissors. In most cases, however, this would not be a long-term solution.
- To initially practise cutting, use materials other than paper. For example, roll out clay or dough snakes and cut off sections with scissors, or practise snipping blades of grass growing in a cup — a mini lawn mower game.
- Introduce cutting with firmer material like old greeting cards, postcards, or light cardboard, as it is easier to control than flimsy paper.
- Tell the child that the scissors (worker) hand *only opens and shuts the scissors* and the paper (helper) hand *only moves the paper.*
- Have the child point their scissors straight to the front of the desk or table.

Helpful hint

- Sometimes a visual cue such as a cup or a glue pot strategically placed on the front of a desk can be helpful in assisting the child to point the scissors to the front as they cut. You can use a visual cue in conjunction with a verbal cue, such as, 'Thumbs on top, thumbs on top, scissors to the glue pot, thumbs on top.'

- Use thick dark lines as guides in beginning scissors tasks. Cue the child to place the blades of the scissors over and under the lines on the paper. The child must keep moving the paper around, so that the cutting line ('road') stays between the blades of the scissors ('car scissors').
- When you have a classroom theme, use themed stories to motivate the children. For example, if the classroom theme is space, tell the children that their scissors are 'space-ships'. Draw a spaceship at the beginning of the line and a planet at the end of the line. Tell them to 'fly' their spaceship on the space road to get to the planet.
- Tell the child that when cutting sharp corners it is like being at a stop sign (you can even place a red dot at this point in initial training). Stop at the corner, keep the scissors facing to the front, and then turn the paper right around before cutting again.
- Gradually decrease the width and darkness of cutting lines.
- When introducing curves or circles, explain that the paper hand will have to turn the paper more frequently to keep up with the scissors hand. Practise cutting out spirals (these can be called space swirls, snakes, seashells, snails, and so on to fit in with your classroom theme).

CHOOSING SCISSORS

One of the easiest to fix but sometimes overlooked reason for poor cutting skills is the actual pair of scissors being used. Some different types of scissors are shown in the picture below.

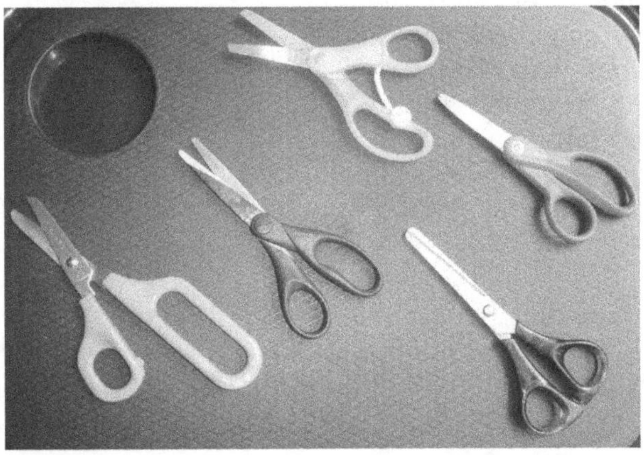

- Be sure to consider right- and left-handed scissors (although many are now for either hand).
- Choose scissors with a shorter blade for beginners. Longer blade scissors are more difficult to control, especially for children with poor hand strength.
- Consider scissors with a single loop for the thumb and a double loop for the index and middle fingers if children cannot use single loop scissors successfully. This will be much easier for many children and could be considered when deciding on the type of scissors to be included in the children's resources lists or classroom 'book packs'.
- Look through therapy and special needs catalogues for dual control training scissors or self-opening scissors if problems persist.

Cutting activities focus points

When you are working on cutting activities with children, the following focus points will assist you in observing that the children are using the correct grasp and cutting action. These focus points can also be found in card format at the beginning of the Cutting activity cards section, for quick reference. A verbal cue or reminder for you to use is given at the end of each focus point.

- **Bilateral coordination**. Ensure the children are using both hands. The worker or dominant hand should be holding the scissors and the helper or non-dominant hand should be holding and turning the paper. **'Two hands'** or **'Helper hand holding the paper'**

- **Elbows by side**. Ensure the worker-hand elbow is relaxed by the side and not held out from the body. **'Elbow in'**

- **Paper rotation**. Ensure the children turn the paper rather than the scissors when they come to a corner or curve. **'Scissors to the front, turn the paper'**

- **Scissors grasp**. For single loop scissors, ensure the thumb is placed in the top loop, the middle finger in the bottom loop, and the index finger supporting underneath. For scissors with a double loop at the bottom, ensure the thumb is placed in the top loop and the index and middle fingers in the bottom loop. **'Check your fingers'** or **'Thumbs on top, thumbs on top, scissors to the glue pot, thumbs on top'**

- **Scissors position**. Ensure the scissors remain pointing to the front. A visual cue such as a glue pot can be used. **'Scissors to the front'** or **'Scissors to the glue pot'**

- **Wrist extension**. During cutting, ensure the wrist is on its side (not turned over with palms down) and slightly extended away from the body (not bent towards the body). **'Wrists up'**

- **Visual focus**. Ensure the children keep their visual focus on the cutting task. Take note of any unusual head positioning to one side. **'Eyes on the job'**

☑ SUPPLIES LIST

For cutting activities

Items from common supplies box

- ☐ Scissors (various types)
- ☐ Corrugated craft card-board
- ☐ Cardboard
- ☐ Glue
- ☐ Paper of varying types and weights
- ☐ Paper plates
- ☐ Coloured pencils, pencils, crayons, markers
- ☐ Permanent marker pen
- ☐ Red pen
- ☐ Sticky tape
- ☐ String
- ☐ Chenille sticks (pipe cleaners)

Additional items

- ☐ Drinking straws
- ☐ Styrofoam
- ☐ Foam craft pieces
- ☐ Bubble wrap
- ☐ Down the Busy Road templates (see resource CD)
- ☐ Perspex® car stamps (available at www.fingergym.info)
- ☐ A Walk in the Park templates (see resource CD)
- ☐ Punch-out flower stamp
- ☐ Any traced work saved from pencil to paper activities
- ☐ Climbing Monkeys templates (see resource CD)
- ☐ Perspex® climbing monkey stamp (available from www.fingergym.resources.com)
- ☐ Puppy template (see resource CD)
- ☐ Train template (see resource CD)
- ☐ Fingergym™ fingers template (see resource CD)
- ☐ Cut Around Egghead template (see resource CD)
- ☐ Cut Around a Snowperson template (see resource CD)
- ☐ Cotton wool balls
- ☐ Make a Fidget Frog™ template (see resource CD)
- ☐ Wallpaper and wallpaper borders
- ☐ Red and green stamp pads
- ☐ Craft materials

Cutting Skills Activities

CARD 1

Cutting Skills Focus Points

- **Bilateral coordination**. Ensure the children are using both hands. The worker or dominant hand should be holding the scissors and the helper or non-dominant hand should be holding and turning the paper. **'Two hands'** or **'Helper hand holding the paper'**
- **Elbows by side**. Ensure the worker-hand elbow is relaxed by the side and not held out from the body. **'Elbow in'**
- **Paper rotation**. Ensure the children turn the paper rather than the scissors when they come to a corner or curve. **'Scissors to the front, turn the paper'**
- **Visual focus**. Ensure the children keep their visual focus on the cutting task. Take note of any unusual head positioning to one side. **'Eyes on the job'**

CARD 2

Cutting Skills Focus Points

- **Scissors grasp**. For single loop scissors, ensure the thumb is placed in the top loop, the middle finger in the bottom loop, and the index finger supporting underneath. For scissors with a double loop at the bottom, ensure the thumb is placed in the top loop and the index and middle fingers in the bottom loop. **'Check your fingers'** or **'Thumbs on top, thumbs on top, scissors to the glue pot, thumbs on top'**
- **Scissors position**. Ensure the scissors remain pointing to the front. A visual cue such as a glue pot can be used. **'Scissors to the front'** or **'Scissors to the glue pot'**
- **Wrist extension**. During cutting, ensure the wrist is on its side (not turned over with palms down) and slightly extended away from the body (not bent towards the body). **'Wrists up'**

CS1

Activity 1: Drinking Straws Cut Up

Tools: Scissors, drinking straws, styrofoam, string, chenille sticks

Action: Cut up straws and stick the pieces into styrofoam to make a pattern, use the pieces for threading onto string or chenille sticks, or use them to create a lovely collage.

Mathematics and Art: Counting, sequencing, patterning

Scissors grasp, wrist extension, bilateral coordination, visual focus

CS2

Activity 2: Ridgy-Didge Cutting

Tools: Scissors, corrugated craft cardboard

Action: Cut along the ridges of corrugated cardboard. Use the strips to make a picture or use them as part of a collage.

Mathematics and Art: Count the number of strips cut.

Scissors grasp, scissors position, wrist extension, elbows by side, bilateral coordination, visual focus

CS3

Activity 3: Foam Cuts

Tools: Scissors, coloured foam craft pieces

Action: Cut across foam pieces. Glue on paper to make a collage.

Mathematics and Art: Counting, sequencing of colours

Scissors grasp, scissors position, wrist extension, elbows by side, bilateral coordination, visual focus

CS4

Activity 4: Cut and Pop

Tools: Scissors, bubble wrap, permanent marker pen

Action: Cut bubble wrap to make it pop.

△ Colour pathway on bubbles to be popped. Cut along specific letters, numbers, or coloured spots.

Hint: A cutting pathway does not have to be in a straight line.

Mathematics and Language: Counting; sequencing; colour, letter, and number identification

Scissors grasp, scissors position, wrist extension, elbows by side, bilateral coordination, visual focus

CS5

Activity 5: Down the Busy Road (Straight Line Cutting)

Tools: Down the Busy Road templates (see resource CD), car stamp, red and green stamp pads, scissors

Action: Use the scissors to cut along the line — the 'busy, straight road'. Start at the green car and stop at the red car (if using car stamps).

△ Draw a longer, thinner line; use regular paper

▽ Draw a shorter, thicker line; use card or firmer paper

Mathematics and Language: Count the number of roads cut, talk about things seen along the way beside a busy road.

Scissors grasp, scissors position, wrist extension, elbows by side, bilateral coordination, visual focus, control of scissors to stop cutting

CS6

Activity 6: Cut the Corner (Curved and Sharp)

Tools: Templates (see resource CD), scissors, red pen or stamping pen

Action: Children use the scissors to cut along the line until they reach the red dot (at the corner), where they then turn the paper and continue cutting.

△ Draw a longer, thinner line; use regular paper

▽ Draw a shorter, thicker line; use card or firmer paper

Language: Talk about turning left and right when you turn a corner

Scissors grasp, scissors position, wrist extension, elbows by side, bilateral coordination, visual focus, paper rotation

CS7

Activity 7: Pizza Cut Up

Tools: Scissors, paper plate or circular piece of cardboard with lines drawn across it to represent pizza pieces, craft materials

Action: Children cut along the lines to make pizza pieces. They then decorate the pieces using bits of craft materials that have been cut up in a prior session.

Language and Mathematics: Discuss cultural foods, sequence of toppings placed on pizza, dividing and fractions

Scissors grasp, scissors position, wrist extension, elbows by side, bilateral coordination, visual focus, paper rotation

CS8

Activity 8: A Walk in the Park (Wavy Line Cutting)

Tools: A Walk in the Park templates (see resource CD), punch out flower stamp for incentives (if needed), scissors

Action: Use the scissors to cut along the winding pathway in the park. Use the punched out shapes as incentives to continue cutting for children who are reluctant or tiring.

△ Draw a longer, thinner line; use regular paper

▽ Draw a shorter, thicker line; use card or firmer paper

Language: Talk about things to see in a park.

Scissors grasp, scissors position, wrist extension, elbows by side, bilateral coordination, visual focus, paper rotation

CS9

Activity 9: Climbing Monkeys (Zigzag Cutting)

Tools: Climbing Monkeys (Zigzag Cutting) templates (see resource CD), perspex® climbing monkey stamp, stamp pads, scissors

Action: The zigzag lines in this activity promote the cutting of sharp angles and turns. Place monkey stamps along the zigzag lines to encourage perseverance. Start at the green monkey and stop at the red one.

Hint: First use the monkey stamp in a stamping activity (similar to SP14 or SP29) with zigzag strips. Use a red spot at the points of the zigzags to help highlight the 'stop and turn' point for the scissors.

△ Draw a longer, thinner line; use regular paper

▽ Draw a shorter, thicker line; use card or firmer paper

Mathematics: Count the monkeys.

Scissors grasp, scissors position, wrist extension, elbows by side, bilateral coordination, visual focus, paper rotation

CS10

Activity 10: Puppy and Train Templates (Group Art)

Tools: Puppy and Train templates (see resource CD), scissors, large sheet of paper, glue

Action: Use the templates and other items from colouring-in books, wall-paper borders, or magazines to cut around and glue onto a large piece of paper to make a Fingergym™ group collage. The group of children will love to display their group efforts to the rest of the class.

Mathematics and Language: Count the number of items, talk about categories of items cut out

Scissors grasp, scissors position, wrist extension, elbows by side, bilateral coordination, visual focus, paper rotation

CS11

Activity 11: Quick Cut Fingers

Tools: Fingergym™ fingers template (see resource CD), scissors

Action: Children cut around the template as many times as they can during the session, aiming for reasonable but not complete accuracy. Use this activity to promote speedy and accurate cutting.

Hint: Make sure you have plenty of supplies for this session, as the children will soon speed up. Use the cut-outs in a collage.

Mathematics: Counting

Scissors grasp, scissors position, wrist extension, elbows by side, bilateral coordination, visual focus, paper rotation, speed with accuracy

CS12

Activity 12: Cut Around Egghead

Tools: Cut Around Egghead template (see resource CD), scissors, glue or sticky tape

Action: Use the scissors to cut neatly around Egghead and to cut out his arms and legs. Children can fan fold the arms and legs before gluing if they are able. Egghead can then be coloured in at another activity station.

Hint: This activity can be done over several sessions. Use as an opportunity to practise collecting and safely storing Egghead parts in the correct place for the next session. Encourage the children to find their Egghead pieces and remember what they had to do and where they were up to in the assembly of their Egghead in the next session. Name or initial each piece.

Mathematics: Count parts, patterning/sequencing

Scissors grasp, scissors position, wrist extension, elbows by side, bilateral coordination, visual focus, paper rotation

CS13

Activity 13: Cut Around a Snowperson

Tools: Cut Around a Snowperson template (see resource CD), scissors, glue, cotton wool

Action: Use the scissors to cut neatly around the snowperson template. Glue on cotton balls to create a picture.

Hint: This activity can be done over several sessions. Use as an opportunity to practise collecting and safely storing parts in the correct place for the next session. Encourage the children to find their snowperson pieces and remember what they had to do and where they were up to in the assembly of their snowperson in the next session. Name or initial each piece.

Mathematics, Language, Art: Count cotton balls, discuss snow topics

Scissors grasp, scissors position, wrist extension, elbows by side, bilateral coordination, visual focus, paper rotation

CS14

Activity 14: Make a Fidget Frog™

Tools: Make a Fidget Frog™ template (see resource CD), scissors, sticky tape, coloured pencils

Action: Use the scissors to cut neatly around the Fidget Frog™ template and also cut along the lines for his arms and legs. Cut out and stick a small strip of paper to Fidget's™ back to make him into a finger puppet.

Hint: This activity can be done over several sessions. Use as an opportunity to practise collecting and safely storing parts in the correct place for the next session. Encourage the children to find their Fidget Frog™ pieces and remember what they had to do and where they were up to in the assembly of Fidget™ in the next session. Name or initial each piece.

Mathematics: Count parts, patterning/sequencing

Scissors grasp, scissors position, wrist extension, elbows by side, bilateral coordination, visual focus, paper rotation

Section C
Appendices, Glossary, References

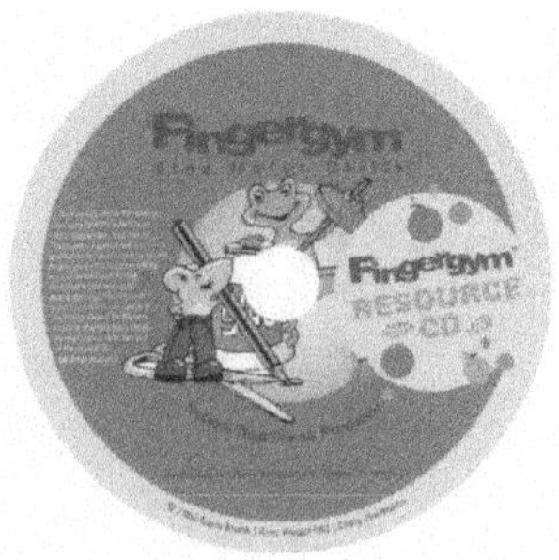 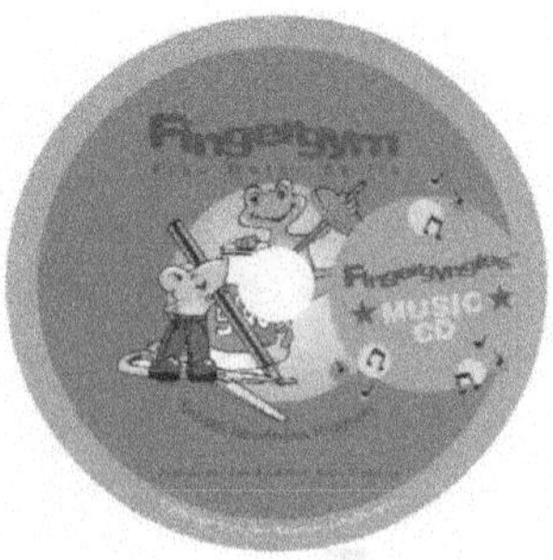

Where are my CDs?

Fingergym was first released in 2006 when CDs were often used to include extra program resources with printed books. Times have changed. Today, many computers exclude CD/DVD players. Therefore we have taken the decision to move the contents of both the Fingergym Resources CD and Fingergym Music CD to secure online digital storage.

Using either the url or QR code links below, the purchaser is permitted to download and save the data and music files on a secure digital storage platform. A permanent licence is granted to the purchaser to print out all the data and play the music files in part or whole on an unlimited basis for the purchaser's own non-profit educational use.

Fingergym Data CD contents

https://sowl.co/bwBF2y

Fingergym Music CD contents

https://sowl.co/zEYut

Appendix A: Resource CD Contents

Folder and File Names Summary

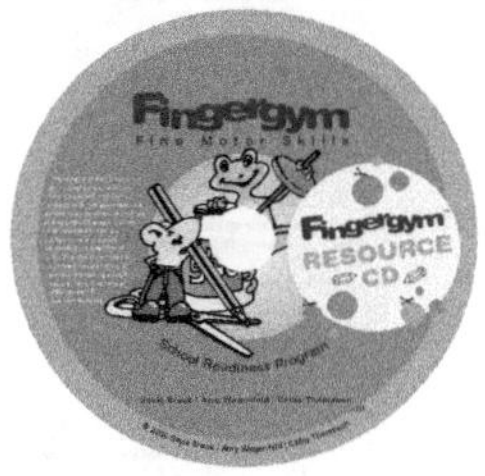

- Read me first.pdf
- Monitoring Forms
  - FORM1.pdf
  - FORM2.pdf
  - FORM3.pdf
  - FORM4.pdf
- Awards and Rewards
  - AWARDS1.pdf
  - AWARDS2.pdf
  - AWARDS3.pdf
  - AWARDS4.pdf
  - AWARDS5.pdf
  - AWARDS6.pdf
  - AWARDS7.pdf
  - AWARDS8.pdf
- Setting Up Tools
  - SET-UP1.pdf
  - SET-UP2.pdf
  - SET-UP3.pdf
  - SET-UP4.pdf
  - SET-UP5.pdf
  - SET-UP6.pdf
  - SET-UP7.pdf
  - SET-UP8.pdf
  - SET-UP9.pdf
  - SET-UP10.pdf
- Activity Templates
  - TEMPLATES1.pdf
  - TEMPLATES2.pdf
  - TEMPLATES3.pdf
  - TEMPLATES4.pdf
  - TEMPLATES5.pdf
  - TEMPLATES6.pdf
  - TEMPLATES7.pdf
  - TEMPLATES8.pdf
  - TEMPLATES9.pdf
  - TEMPLATES10.pdf
  - TEMPLATES11.pdf
  - TEMPLATES12.pdf
  - TEMPLATES13.pdf
  - TEMPLATES14.pdf
  - TEMPLATES15.pdf
  - TEMPLATES16.pdf
  - TEMPLATES17.pdf
  - TEMPLATES18.pdf
  - TEMPLATES19.pdf
  - TEMPLATES20.pdf
  - TEMPLATES21.pdf
  - TEMPLATES22.pdf
  - TEMPLATES23.pdf
  - TEMPLATES24.pdf
  - TEMPLATES25.pdf
  - TEMPLATES26.pdf
  - TEMPLATES27.pdf
  - TEMPLATES28.pdf
  - TEMPLATES29.pdf
  - TEMPLATES30.pdf
  - TEMPLATES31.pdf
  - TEMPLATES32.pdf
  - TEMPLATES33.pdf
  - TEMPLATES34.pdf
  - TEMPLATES35.pdf
- Customisable Documents
  - AWARDS.doc
  - LETTER1.doc
  - LETTER2.doc
  - LETTER3.doc

Thumbnail images of these files follow, also to help you easily find the file or files you are looking for.

Monitoring Forms

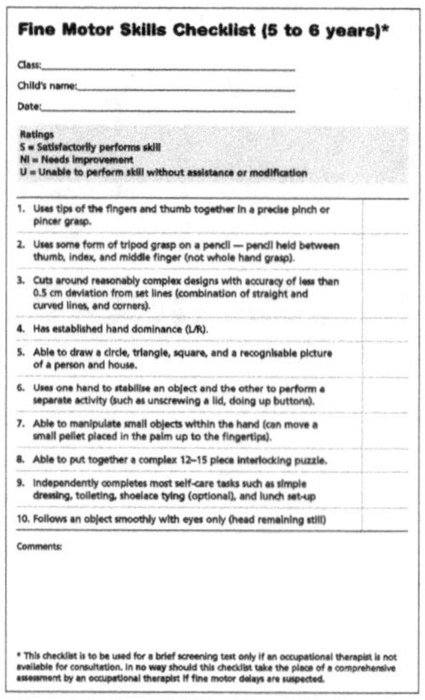

Fine Motor Skills Checklist (5 to 6 years)*

Class:__________

Child's name:__________

Date:__________

Ratings
S = Satisfactorily performs skill
NI = Needs improvement
U = Unable to perform skill without assistance or modification

1. Uses tips of the fingers and thumb together in a precise pinch or pincer grasp.
2. Uses some form of tripod grasp on a pencil — pencil held between thumb, index, and middle finger (not whole hand grasp).
3. Cuts around reasonably complex designs with accuracy of less than 0.5 cm deviation from set lines (combination of straight and curved lines, and corners).
4. Has established hand dominance (L/R).
5. Able to draw a circle, triangle, square, and a recognisable picture of a person and house.
6. Uses one hand to stabilise an object and the other to perform a separate activity (such as unscrewing a lid, doing up buttons).
7. Able to manipulate small objects within the hand (can move a small pellet placed in the palm up to the fingertips).
8. Able to put together a complex 12–15 piece interlocking puzzle.
9. Independently completes most self-care tasks such as simple dressing, toileting, shoelace tying (optional), and lunch set-up
10. Follows an object smoothly with eyes only (head remaining still)

Comments:

* This checklist is to be used for a brief screening test only if an occupational therapist is not available for consultation. In no way should this checklist take the place of a comprehensive assessment by an occupational therapist if fine motor delays are suspected.

Fine Motor Skills Checklist (5 to 6 years)
FORM1.pdf

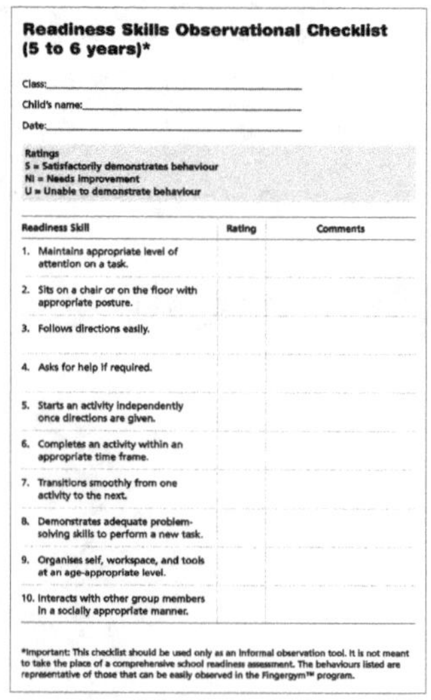

Readiness Skills Observational Checklist (5 to 6 years)*

Class:__________

Child's name:__________

Date:__________

Ratings
S = Satisfactorily demonstrates behaviour
NI = Needs improvement
U = Unable to demonstrate behaviour

Readiness Skill	Rating	Comments
1. Maintains appropriate level of attention on a task.		
2. Sits on a chair or on the floor with appropriate posture.		
3. Follows directions easily.		
4. Asks for help if required.		
5. Starts an activity independently once directions are given.		
6. Completes an activity within an appropriate time frame.		
7. Transitions smoothly from one activity to the next.		
8. Demonstrates adequate problem-solving skills to perform a new task.		
9. Organises self, workspace, and tools at an age-appropriate level.		
10. Interacts with other group members in a socially appropriate manner.		

*Important: This checklist should be used only as an informal observation tool. It is not meant to take the place of a comprehensive school readiness assessment. The behaviours listed are representative of those that can be easily observed in the Fingergym™ program.

Readiness Skills Observational Checklist (5 to 6 years)
FORM2.pdf

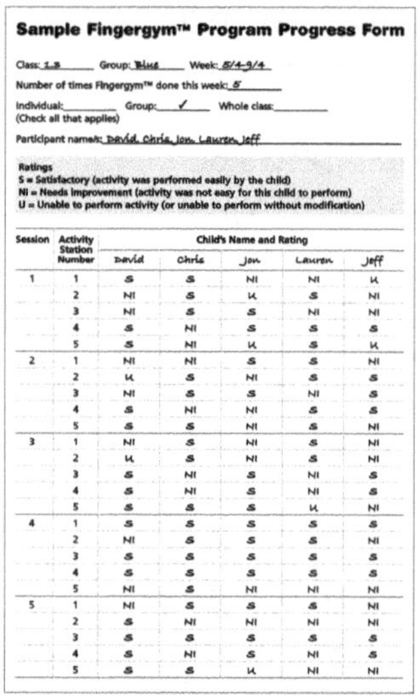

Sample Fingergym™ Program Progress Form

Class: 1.3 Group: Blue Week: 5/4-9/4

Number of times Fingergym™ done this week: 5

Individual:_____ Group: ✓ Whole class:_____
(Check all that applies)

Participant name/s: David, Chris, Jon, Lauren, Jeff

Ratings
S = Satisfactory (activity was performed easily by the child)
NI = Needs improvement (activity was not easy for this child to perform)
U = Unable to perform activity (or unable to perform without modification)

Session	Activity Station Number	Child's Name and Rating				
		David	Chris	Jon	Lauren	Jeff
1	1	S	S	NI	NI	U
	2	NI	S	U	S	NI
	3	NI	S	S	NI	NI
	4	S	NI	S	S	S
	5	S	NI	U	S	U
2	1	NI	NI	S	S	NI
	2	U	S	NI	S	S
	3	NI	S	S	NI	S
	4	S	NI	NI	S	S
	5	S	S	NI	S	NI
3	1	NI	S	NI	S	NI
	2	U	S	NI	S	NI
	3	S	NI	S	NI	S
	4	S	NI	S	NI	S
	5	S	S	S	U	NI
4	1	S	S	S	S	S
	2	NI	S	S	S	NI
	3	S	S	S	S	S
	4	S	S	S	S	S
	5	NI	S	NI	NI	NI
5	1	NI	S	S	S	NI
	2	S	NI	NI	NI	NI
	3	S	S	S	S	S
	4	S	NI	S	NI	S
	5	S	S	U	NI	NI

Sample Fingergym™ Program Progress Form
FORM3.pdf

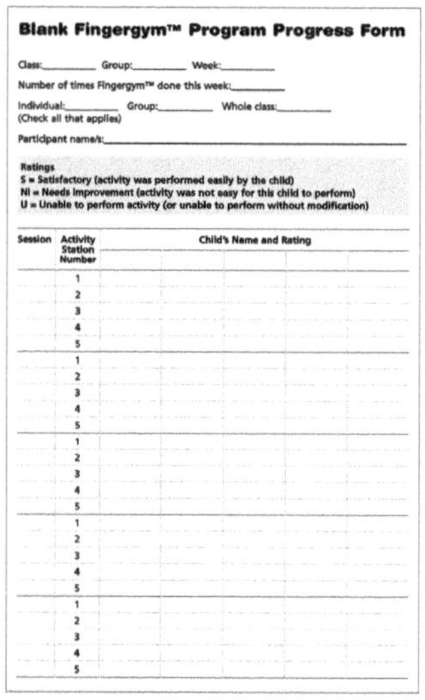

Blank Fingergym™ Program Progress Form

Class:_____ Group:_____ Week:_____

Number of times Fingergym™ done this week:_____

Individual:_____ Group:_____ Whole class:_____
(Check all that applies)

Participant name/s:__________

Ratings
S = Satisfactory (activity was performed easily by the child)
NI = Needs improvement (activity was not easy for this child to perform)
U = Unable to perform activity (or unable to perform without modification)

Session	Activity Station Number	Child's Name and Rating				
	1					
	2					
	3					
	4					
	5					
	1					
	2					
	3					
	4					
	5					
	1					
	2					
	3					
	4					
	5					
	1					
	2					
	3					
	4					
	5					
	1					
	2					
	3					
	4					
	5					

Blank Fingergym™ Program Progress Form
FORM4.pdf

Awards and Rewards

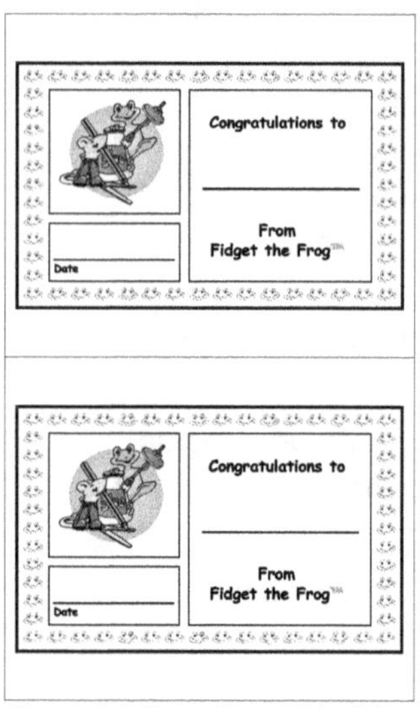

Congratulations From Fidget the Frog™
AWARDS1.pdf

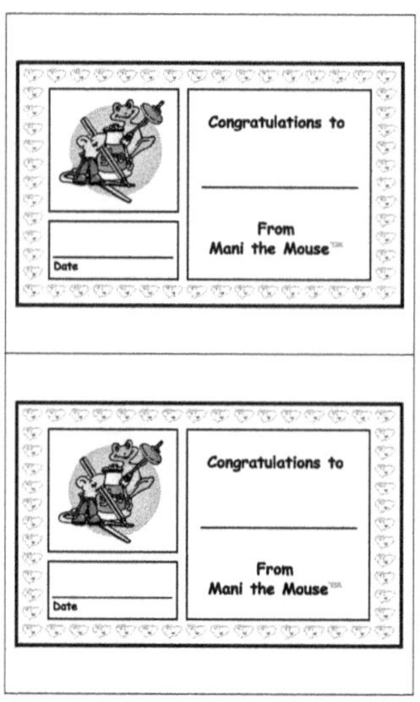

Congratulation From Mani the Mouse™
AWARDS2.pdf

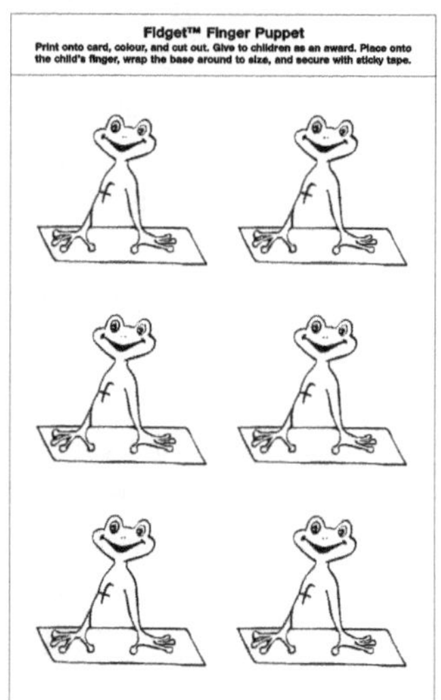

Fidget™ Finger Puppet
AWARDS3.pdf

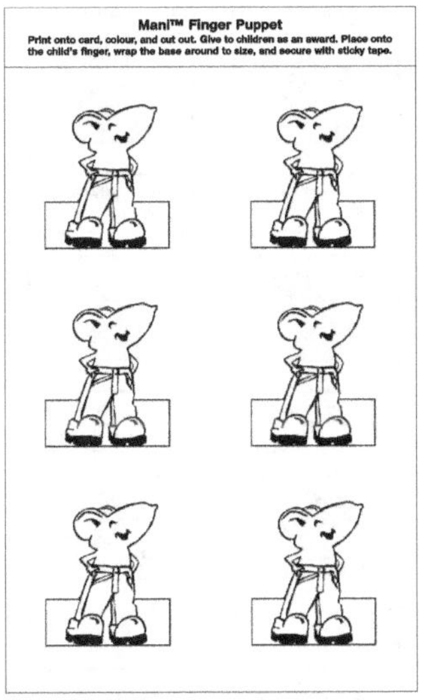

Mani™ Finger Puppet
AWARDS4.pdf

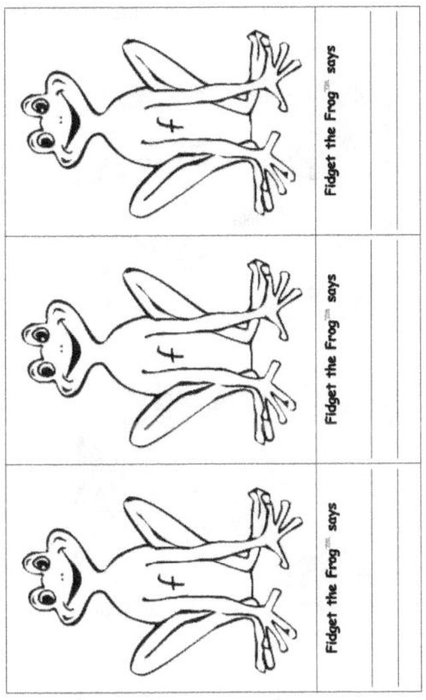

Fidget™ says
AWARDS5.pdf

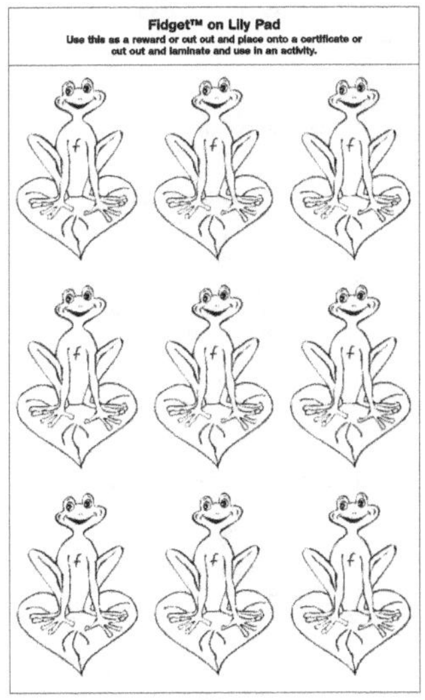

Fidget™ on Lily Pad
AWARDS6.pdf

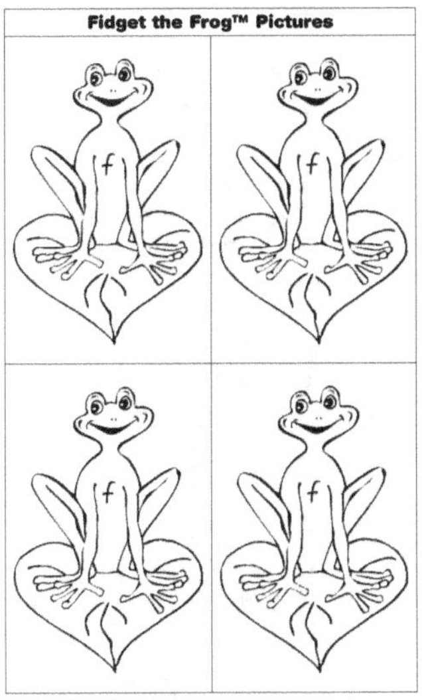

Fidget the Frog™ Pictures
AWARDS7.pdf

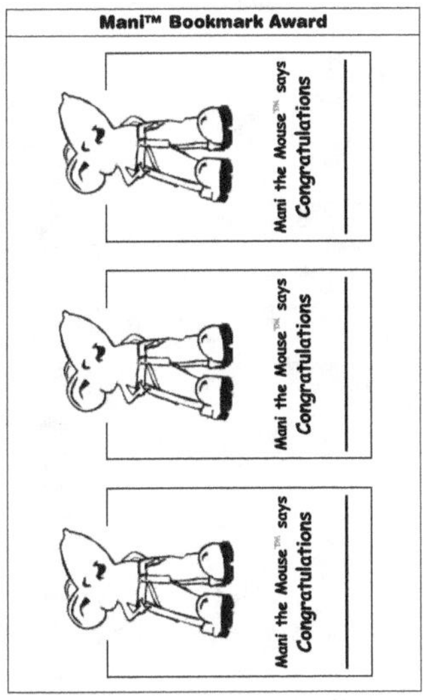

Mani™ Bookmark Award
AWARDS8.pdf

Setting Up Tools

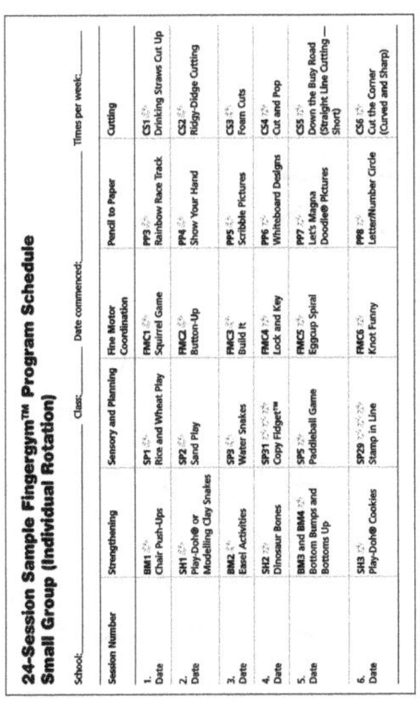

24-Session Sample Fingergym™ Program Schedule
SET-UP1.pdf

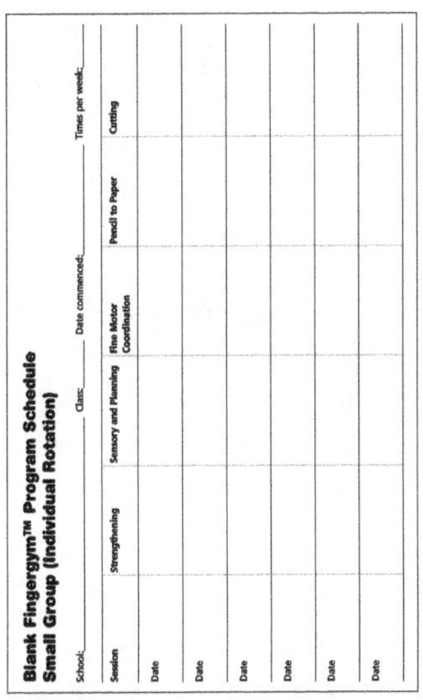

Blank Fingergym™ Program Schedule
SET-UP2.pdf

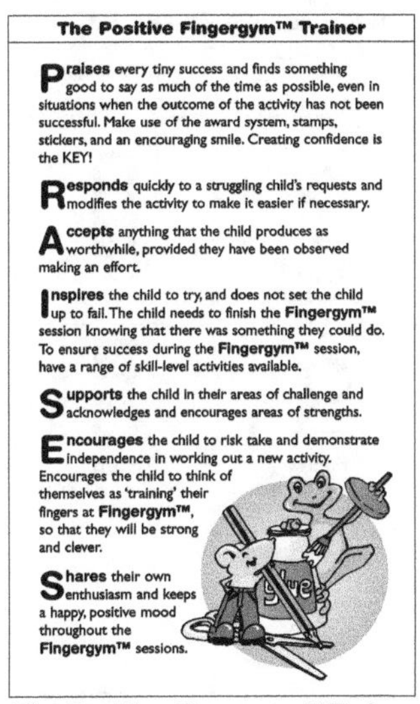

The Positive Fingergym™ Trainer

Praises every tiny success and finds something good to say as much of the time as possible, even in situations when the outcome of the activity has not been successful. Make use of the award system, stamps, stickers, and an encouraging smile. Creating confidence is the KEY!

Responds quickly to a struggling child's requests and modifies the activity to make it easier if necessary.

Accepts anything that the child produces as worthwhile, provided they have been observed making an effort.

Inspires the child to try, and does not set the child up to fail. The child needs to finish the **Fingergym™** session knowing that there was something they could do. To ensure success during the **Fingergym™** session, have a range of skill-level activities available.

Supports the child in their areas of challenge and acknowledges and encourages areas of strengths.

Encourages the child to risk take and demonstrate independence in working out a new activity. Encourages the child to think of themselves as 'training' their fingers at **Fingergym™**, so that they will be strong and clever.

Shares their own enthusiasm and keeps a happy, positive mood throughout the **Fingergym™** sessions.

The Positive Fingergym™ Trainer
SET-UP3.pdf

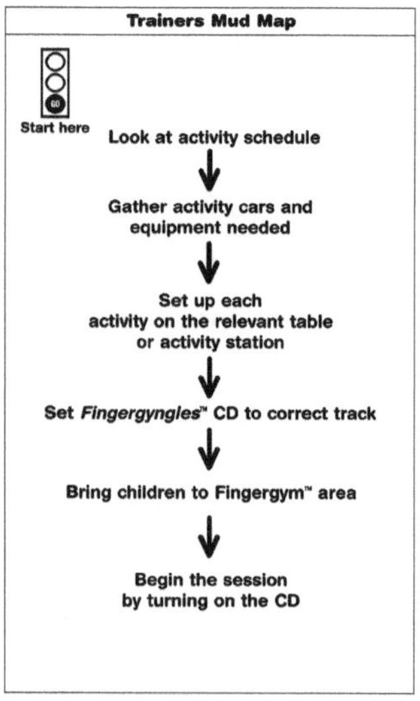

Trainers Mud Map
SET-UP4.pdf

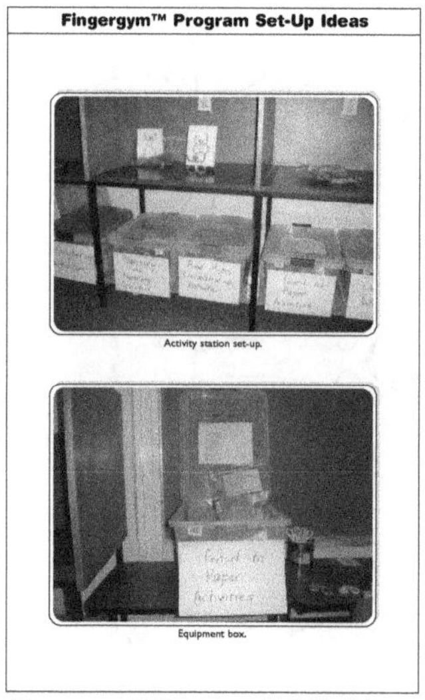

Fingergym™ Program Set-Up Ideas
SET-UP5.pdf

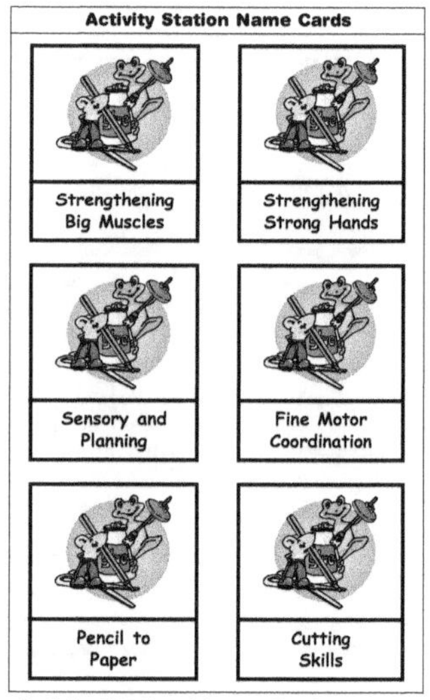

Activity Station Name Cards
SET-UP6.pdf

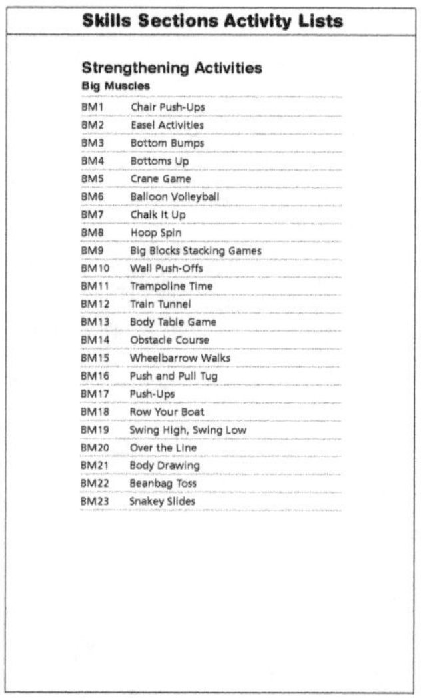

Skill Sections Activity Lists
SET-UP7.pdf

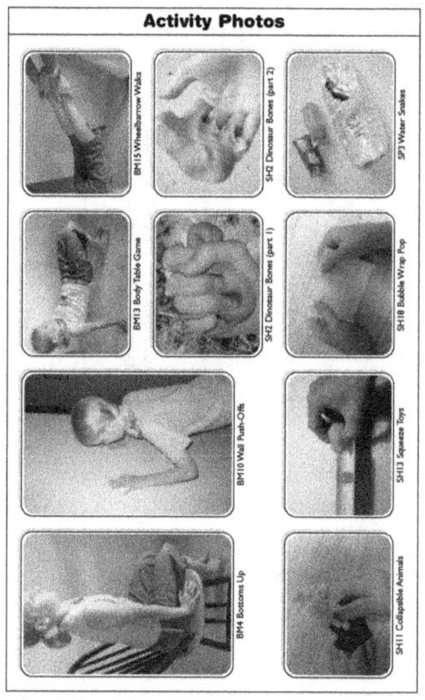

Activity Photos
SET-UP8.pdf

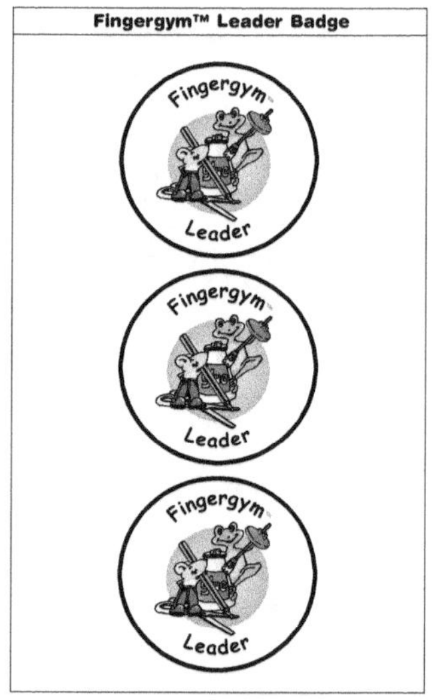

Fingergym™ Leader Badge
SET-UP9.pdf

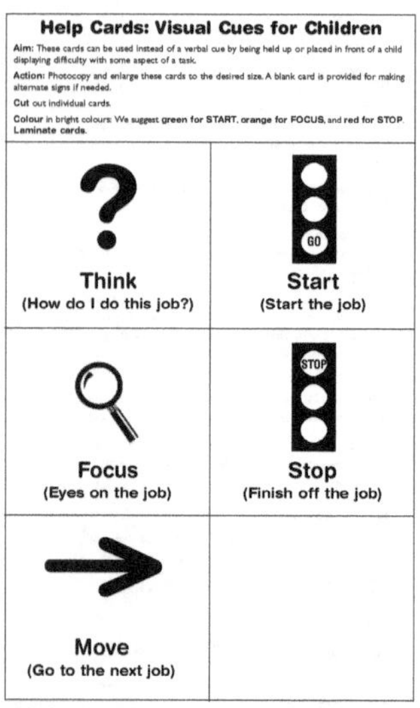

Help Cards: Visual Cues for Children
SET-UP10.pdf

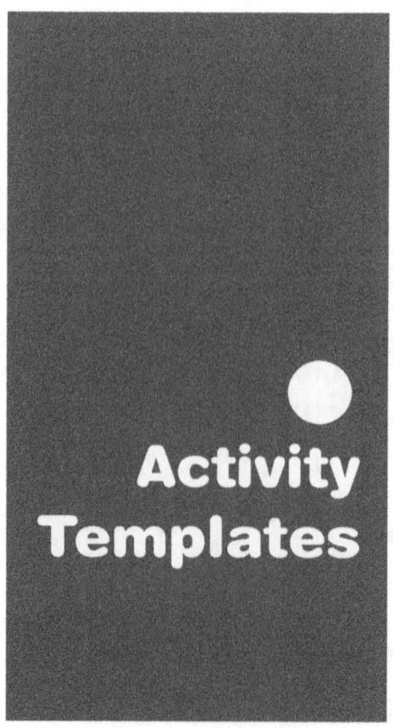

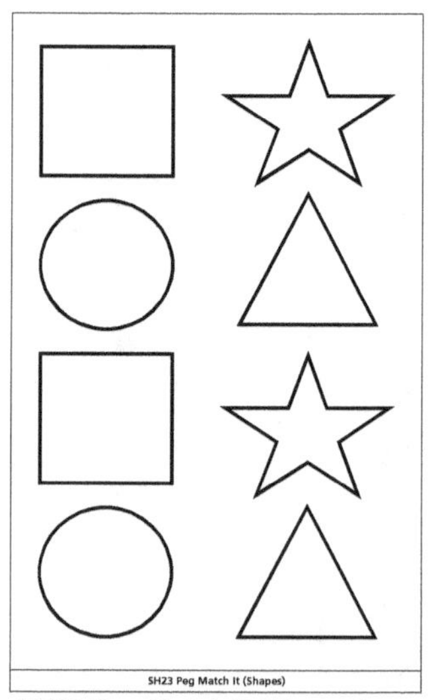

SH23 Peg Match It (Shapes)
TEMPLATES1.pdf

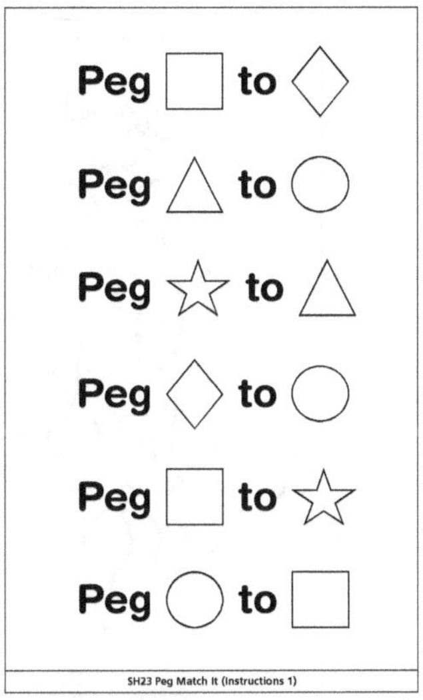

SH23 Peg Match It (Instructions 1)
TEMPLATES2.pdf

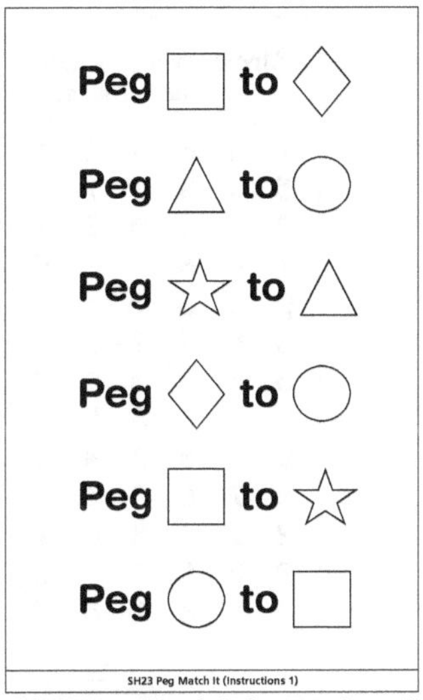

SH23 Peg Match It (Instructions 2)
TEMPLATES3.pdf

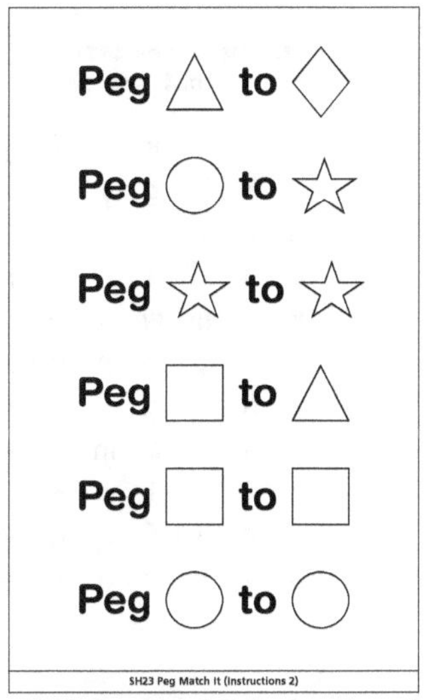

SH23 Peg Match It (Instructions 3)
TEMPLATES4.pdf

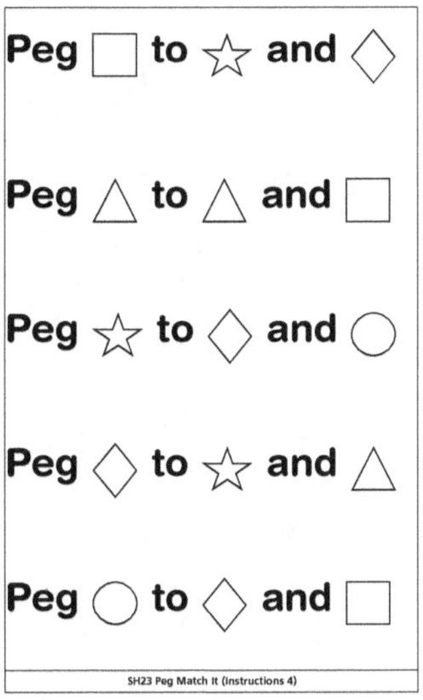

SH23 Peg Match It (Instructions 4)
TEMPLATES5.pdf

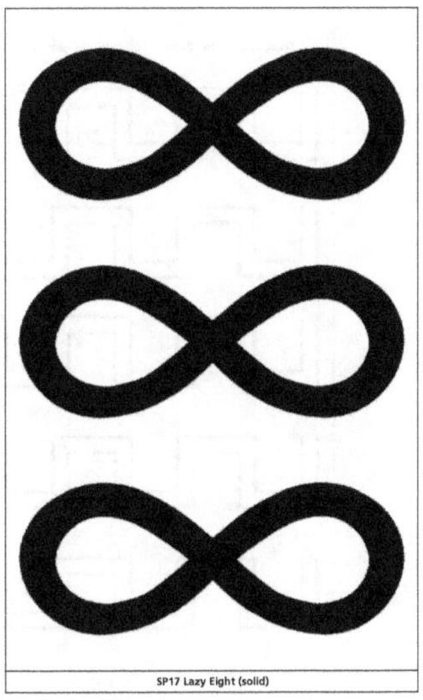

SP17 Lazy Eight (solid)
TEMPLATES6.pdf

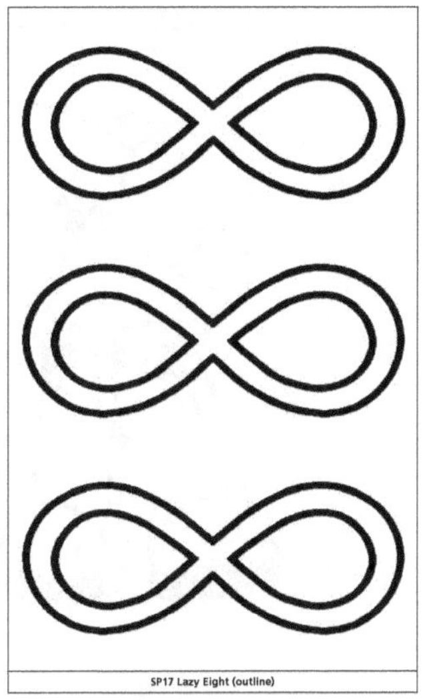

SP17 Lazy Eight (outline)
TEMPLATES7.pdf

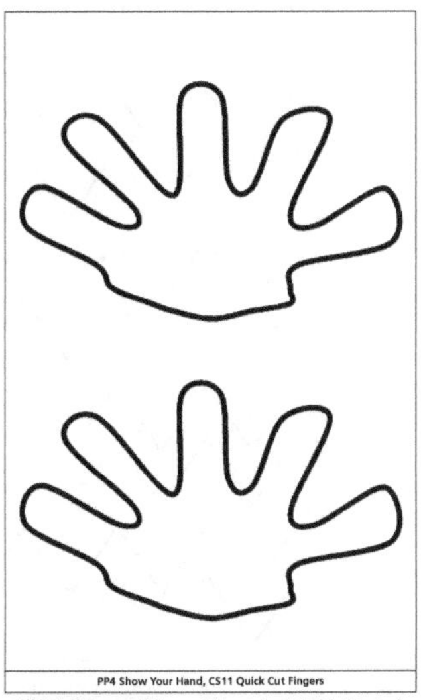

PP4 Show Your Hand; CS11 Quick Cut Fingers
TEMPLATES8.pdf

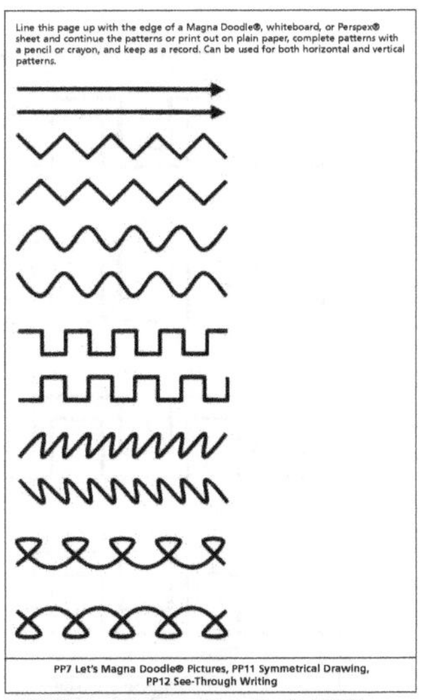

PP7 Lets Magna Doodle ®, PP11 Symmetrical Drawing, PP12 See-Through Writing
TEMPLATES9.pdf

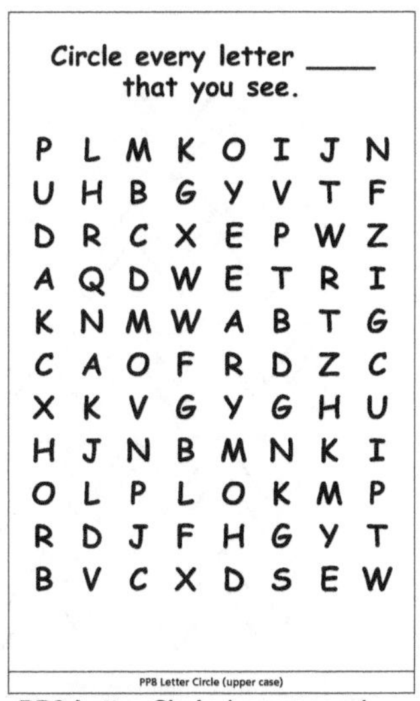

PP8 Letter Circle (upper case)
TEMPLATES10.pdf

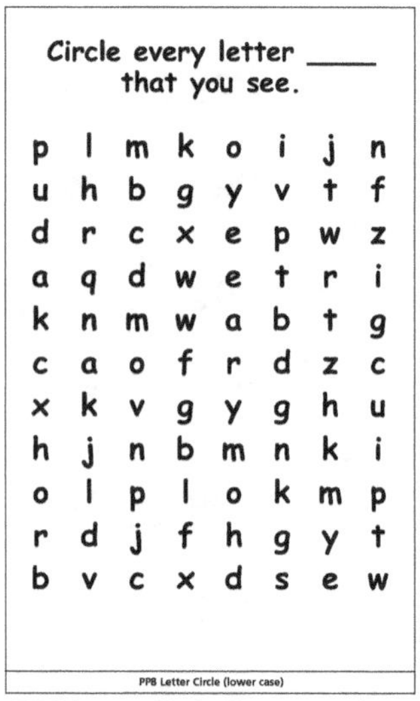

PP8 Letter Circle (lower case)
TEMPLATES11.pdf

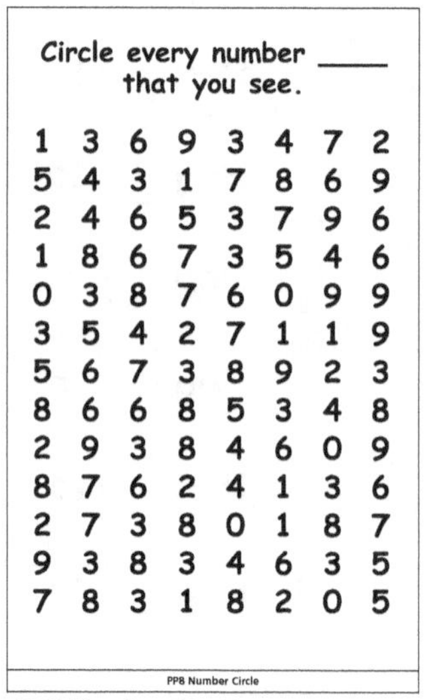

PP8 Number Circle
TEMPLATES12.pdf

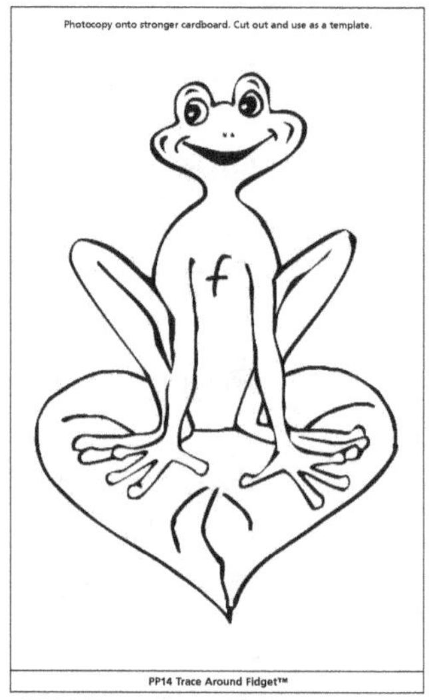

PP14 Trace Around Fidget™
TEMPLATES13.pdf

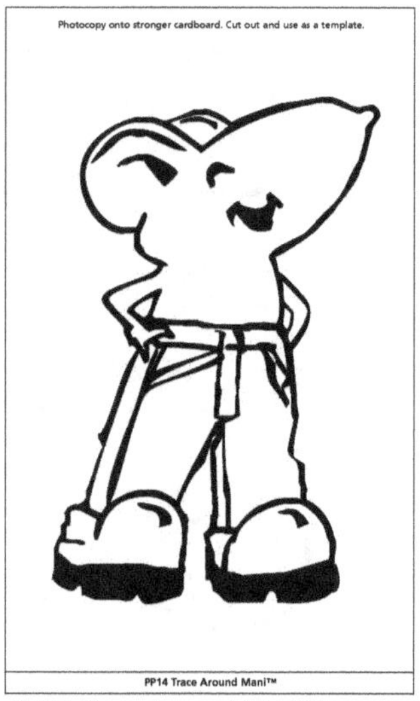

PP14 Trace Around Mani™
TEMPLATES14.pdf

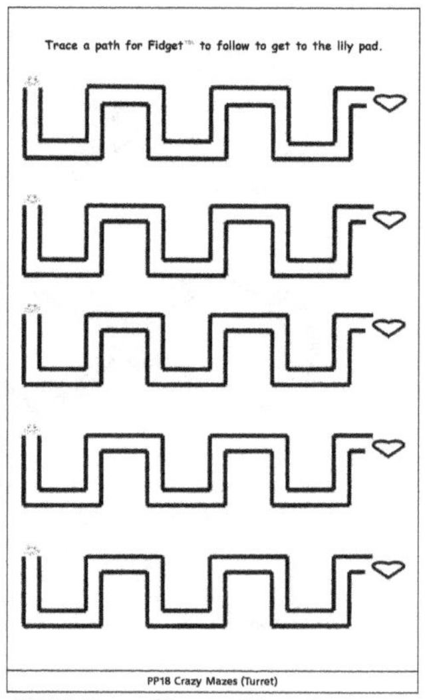

PP18 Crazy Mazes (Turret)
TEMPLATES15.pdf

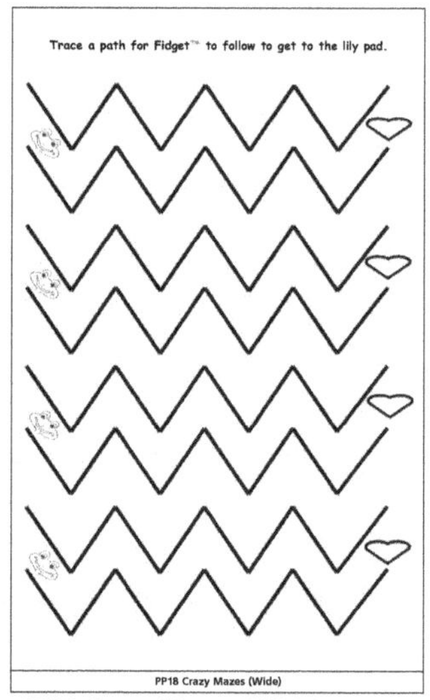

PP18 Crazy Mazes (Wide)
TEMPLATES16.pdf

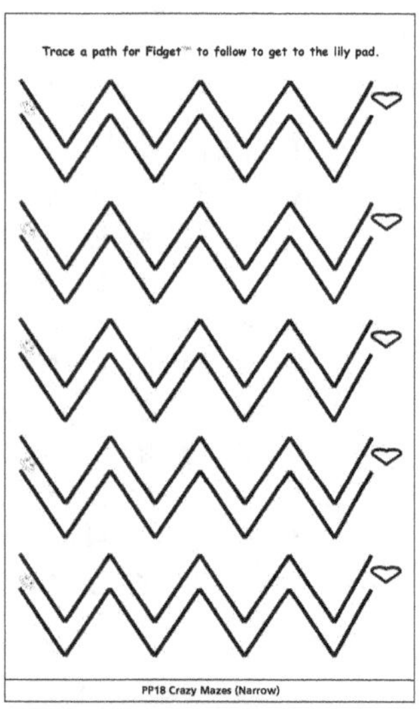

PP18 Crazy Mazes (Narrow)
TEMPLATES17.pdf

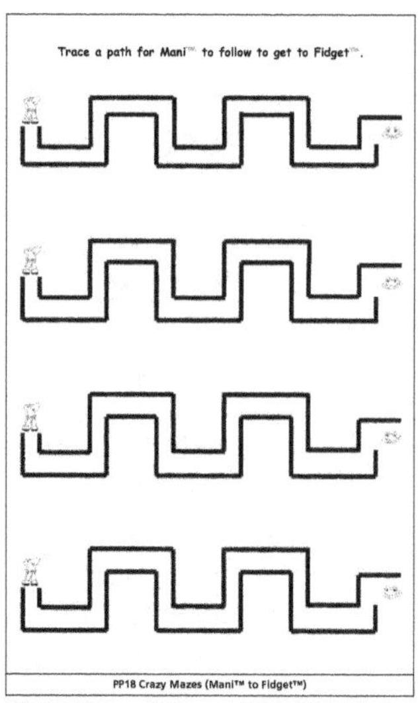

PP18 Crazy Mazes (Mani™ to Fidget™)
TEMPLATES18.pdf

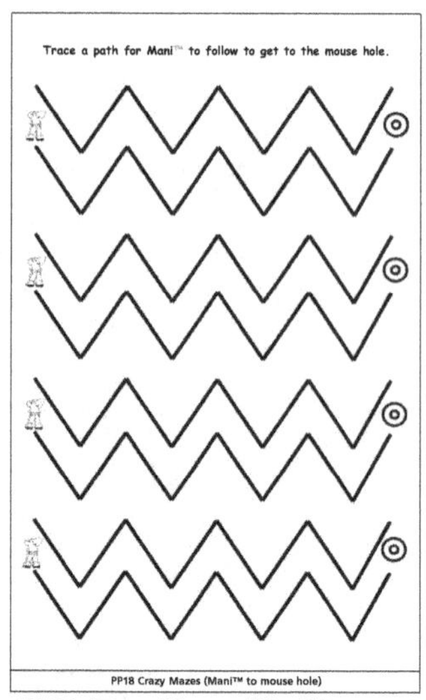

PP18 Crazy Mazes (Mani™ to mouse hole)
TEMPLATES19.pdf

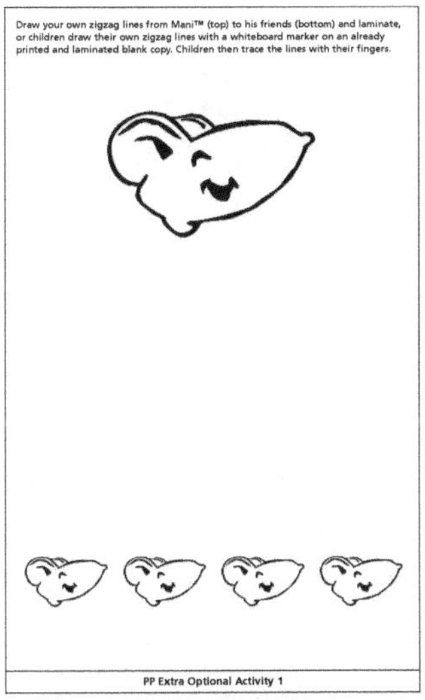

PP Extra Optional Activity
TEMPLATES20.pdf

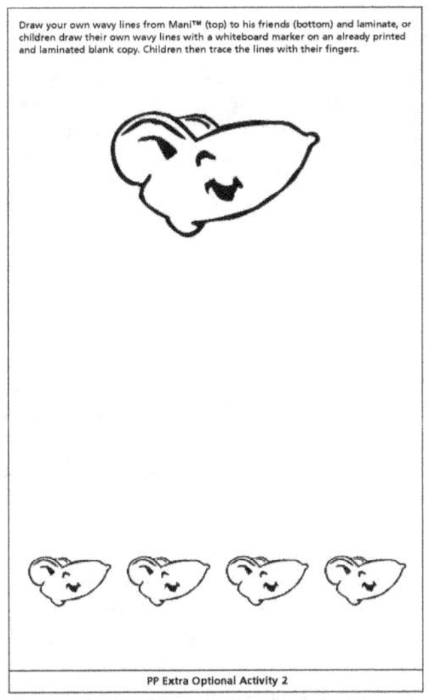

PP Extra Optional Activity 2
TEMPLATES21.pdf

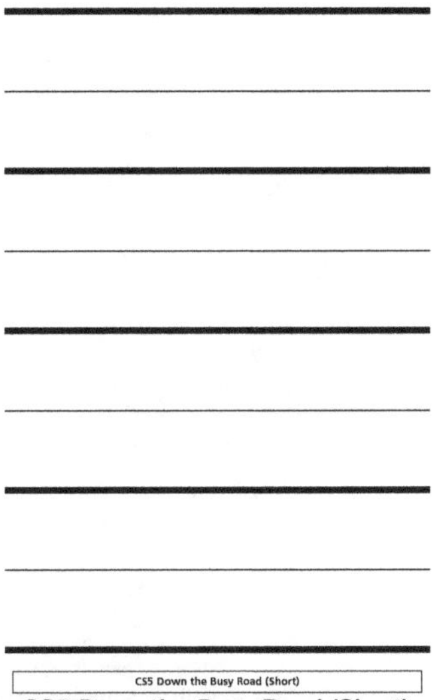

CS5 Down the Busy Road (Short)
TEMPLATES22.pdf

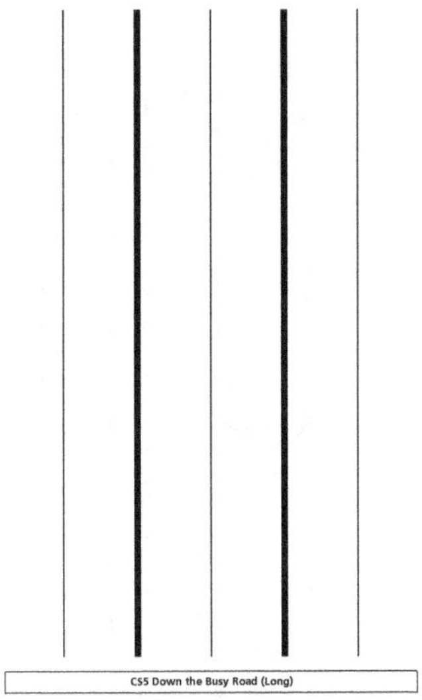

CS5 Down the Busy Road (Long)
TEMPLATES23.pdf

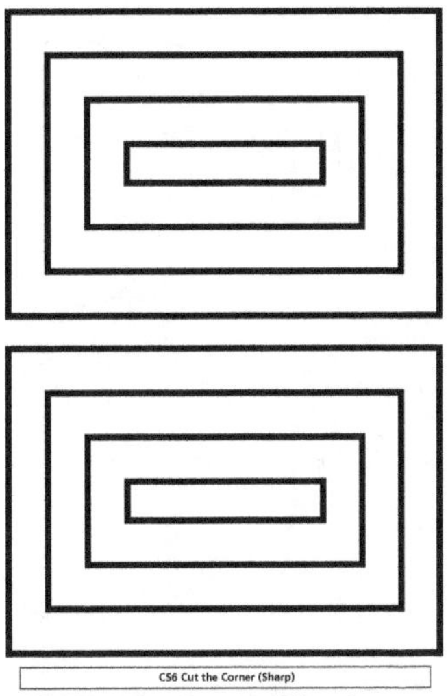

CS6 Cut the Corner (Sharp)
TEMPLATES24.pdf

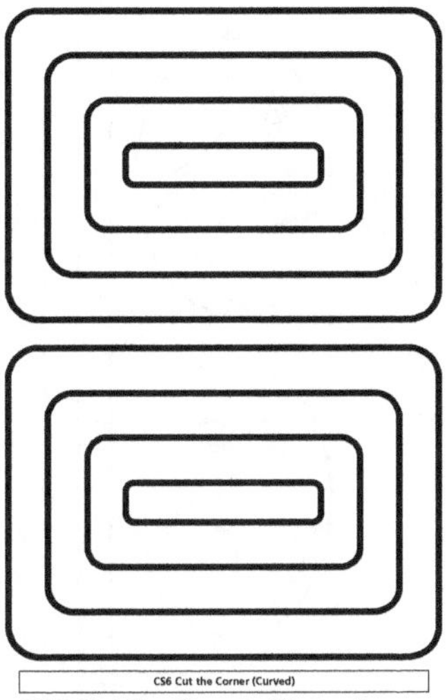

CS6 Cut the Corner (Curved)
TEMPLATES25.pdf

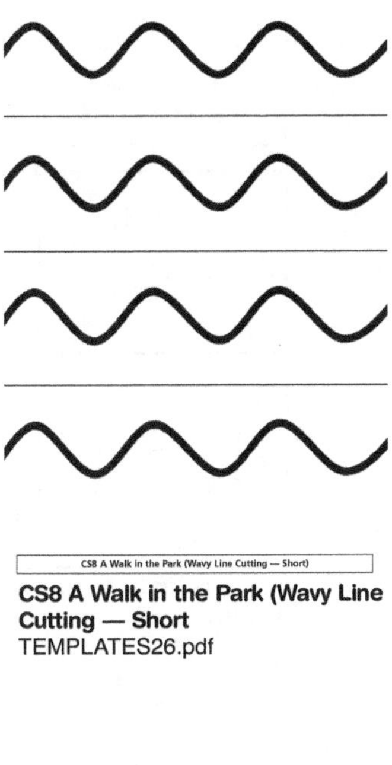

CS8 A Walk in the Park (Wavy Line Cutting — Short
TEMPLATES26.pdf

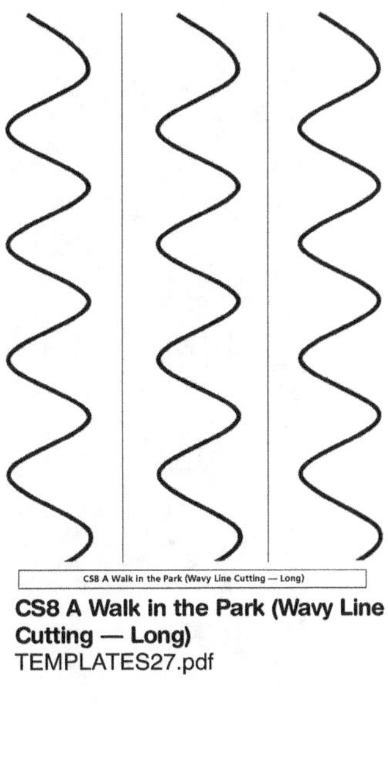

CS8 A Walk in the Park (Wavy Line Cutting — Long)
TEMPLATES27.pdf

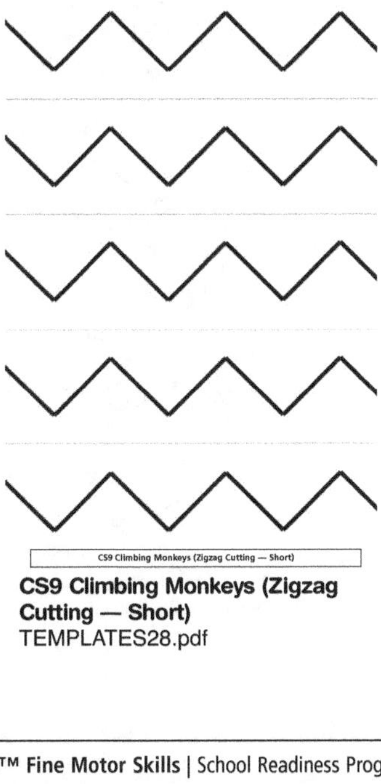

CS9 Climbing Monkeys (Zigzag Cutting — Short)
TEMPLATES28.pdf

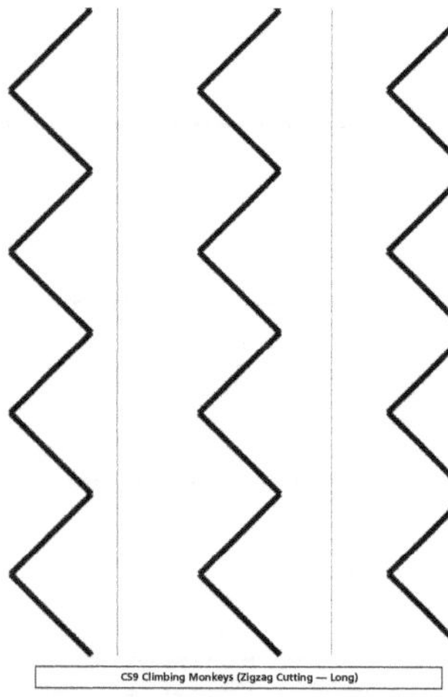

CS9 Climbing Monkeys (Zigzag Cutting — Long)
TEMPLATES29.pdf

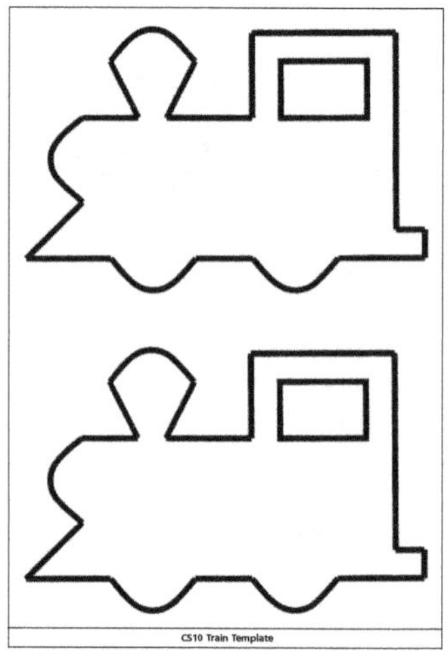

CS10 Train Template
TEMPLATES30.pdf

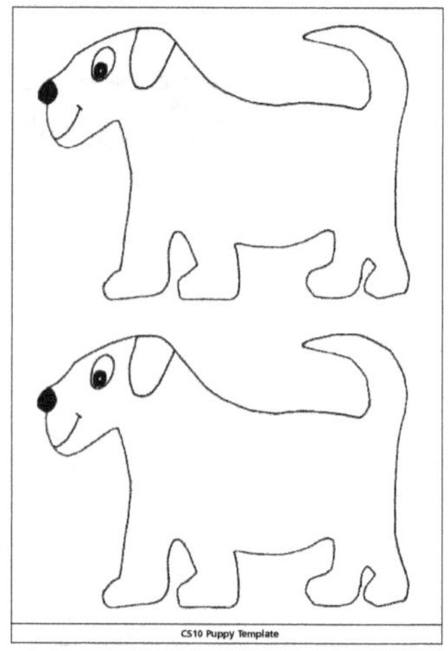

CS10 Puppy Template
TEMPLATES31.pdf

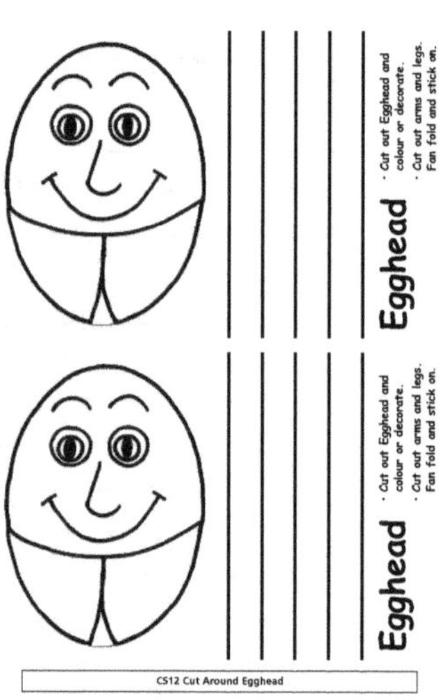

CS12 Cut Around Egghead
TEMPLATES32.pdf

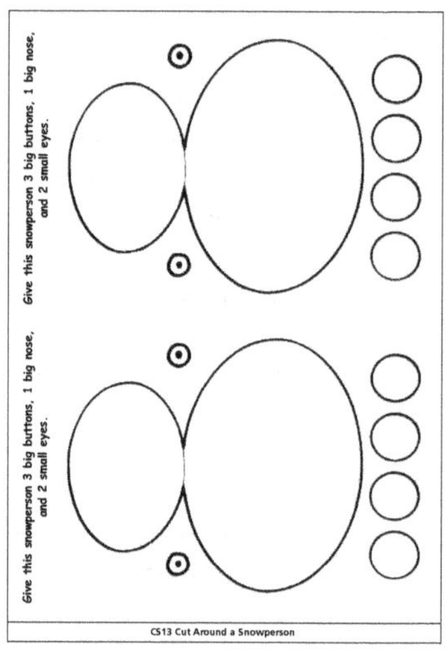

CS13 Cut Around a Snowperson
TEMPLATES33.pdf

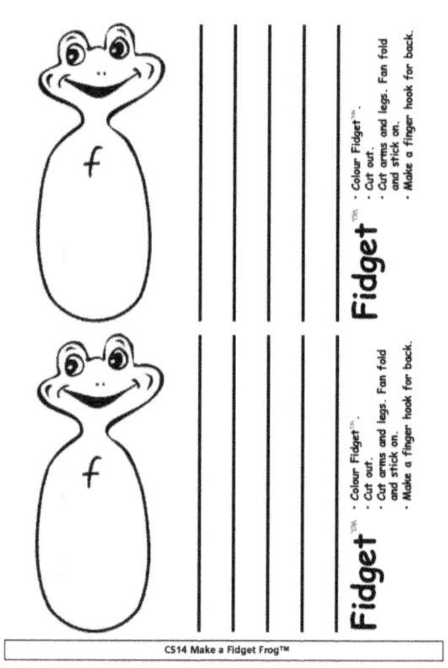

CS14 Make a Fidget Frog™
TEMPLATES34.pdf

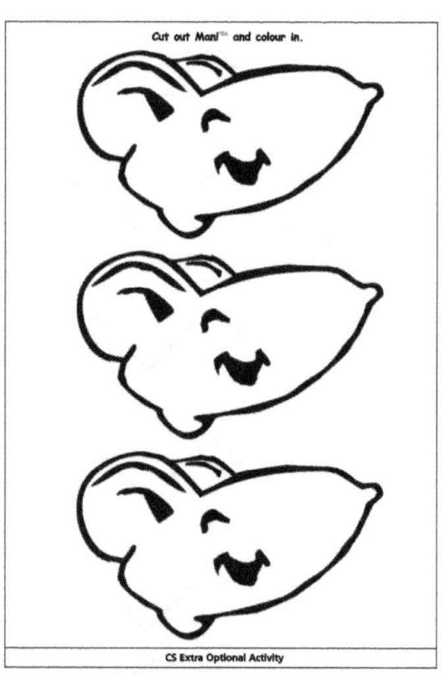

CS Extra Optional Activity
TEMPLATES35.pdf

Customisable Documents

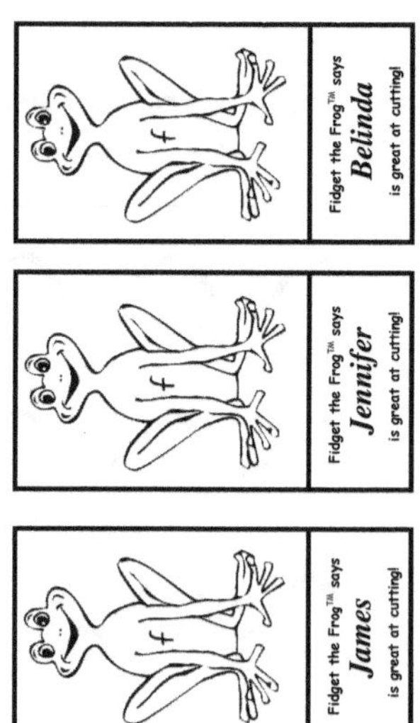

Fidget the Frog™ says
AWARDS.doc

Parent Information Letter

Dear Parents and Caregivers,

RE: The Fingergym™ Fine Motor Skills School Readiness Program

Your child ______________________________ has been selected to take part in our Fingergym™ program.

Children who benefit from participating in Fingergym™ are those who need a little extra practice with fine motor activities such as cutting, pencil skills, manipulating small objects, and activities that are designed to strengthen shoulder, hand, and finger muscles.

Fingergym™ can also be of benefit to children who need help in other areas, such as:

- organising themselves and their possessions
- starting and finishing tasks
- confidence to have a go
- asking for help when needing it
- following instructions.

Fingergym™ sessions are of approximately 15 minutes' duration and will be run __________ times each week.

If you have any questions about the Fingergym™ program, or you would like to see the program in action or volunteer your help, please don't hesitate to contact __________________________'s class teacher.

Yours sincerely,

____

Parent Information Letter
LETTER1.doc

Parent Permission Letter

Dear Parents and Caregivers,

As part of this year's classroom experience, we will be implementing an exciting fine motor skills program called **Fingergym™ Fine Motor Skills School Readiness Program**. This program is designed to develop your child's hand and finger skills (fine motor skills) through various activities. Fingergym™ will provide your child with extra opportunities to strengthen their muscles, develop their senses, coordinate their fingers, and practice drawing, writing, cutting, and using other school tools.

It will also be of benefit to children who need help in other areas such as organising themselves and their possessions, starting and finishing tasks, developing confidence, asking for help when needed, and following instructions.

Fingergym™ sessions will run ______________________ time/s a week on ____ (days).

Please sign below and return to me by __________ (date) to show that ____________________ (child's name) has your permission to participate in this program. Please do not hesitate to contact me with any questions you have regarding this fun and exciting program.

____________________ ____________________
Child's Name Class

has my permission to participate in the Fingergym™ program.

____________________________ ____________________
Parent's or Caregiver's Signature Date

Parent Permission Letter
LETTER2.doc

Volunteer Request Letter

Dear Parents, Grandparents, Caregivers, and Other Interested Volunteers,

I am seeking out a team of dedicated and enthusiastic volunteers to help run a new program called **Fingergym™ Fine Motor Skills School Readiness Program**.

Volunteering will involve helping small groups of children develop better use of their hands for cutting, pencil skills, and much more by strengthening their finger and hand muscles through fun, fine motor activities.

I will be running this program on ________________________ (day/s of week) between ____ (time).

If you can also help with more than running the program, such as helping me keep the activities neat and orderly, and the supplies well stocked, it would also be greatly appreciated.

If you are interested, please fill out the section below and return this form to me by ________________________________ (date).

Thank you so much,

____

I would love to help with the Fingergym™ program by (tick applicable boxes):

- ☐ assisting in the classroom to help run the program
- ☐ keeping the activities in good order in the classroom/restocking supplies.

Days available ____

Name ____

Phone number and/or e-mail address ______________________________

Volunteer Request Letter
LETTER3.doc

Appendix B: Field Trials

'Every day the children would ask, "Is this a Fingergym™ day?", "Can we do Fingergym™?" Such enthusiasm!'

We invited 11 experienced teachers / teacher aides from the Brisbane, Australia area to participate in a four- to eight-week trial of the Fingergym™ program in their school. The trials were not intended to be clinical trials of improvements noted in students' fine motor skills, as benefits from practising fine motor and other related skills have been reported elsewhere. Rather, the purpose of the trials was to receive feedback on the perceived value and feasibility of a fine motor skills program developed for educators of young children.

Sixty-four per cent of the teachers / teacher aides in the trials reported having 16 or more years of classroom experience, and 36% reported having 11 to 15 years of classroom experience. This group represented teachers / teacher aides from preschool, Year 1, Year 3, and special needs classrooms. The average classroom size was 25.3 students. Along with typically developing children, teachers / teacher aides reported that children with autistic spectrum disorders (ASD), intellectual impairment (II), developmental disabilities (DD), speech / language disorders, learning disabilities (LD), attention-deficit disorder (ADD) or attention-deficit / hyperactivity disorder (ADHD), English as a second language (ESL), and unspecified special needs were also enrolled in their classrooms. Teachers / teacher aides also indicated that collectively, 3% of the children in their classroom received occupational therapy services.

Every teacher / teacher aide reported positive and enthusiastic comments about the program, and all indicated that they would, budget permitting, purchase the program and unequivocally recommend it to other teachers and educators. Some of the comments about the program included:

> 'They [children] loved it — looking forward to every Tuesday afternoon. I would love to incorporate this into our routine next year!'
>
> 'Saw improvements in a short time.'
>
> 'Good routine for intellectually impaired or special needs students.'
>
> 'Children enjoyed the activities and it put a focus on writing.'
>
> 'It is an effective, positive program that shows children that we all improve with practice. That is important to learn!'

Comments about what the children who participated in the trial programs thought included:

> 'Loved it! Asked when next session was — laughed during activities — saw it as a "fun" activity not a learning activity.'
>
> 'Children loved it, very much so.'
>
> '[The children] Asked to keep doing [the program] after we had finished.'

In terms of the small group or whole class program trials, of seven who participated, 56% of the teachers/teacher aides chose to implement it two times a week, 36% once a week, and 1% three times a week. Teachers/teacher aides reported that aides, learning support teachers, and volunteers helped them run, obtain materials, and organise the program. One concern expressed about materials was that consistent with most activity programs, materials could become costly over time, but with proper budgeting and parental support that obstacle was far surpassed by the worth and value of the program.

Seventy-three per cent of the teachers/teacher aides reported that the introductory, theory-based chapters were helpful, and that organising the activities by categories was also a positive feature of the program.

For those teachers who reported setting goals for the participants, strong hands activities (from the strengthening activities section), touch and tell activities — arm, finger, and hand awareness (from the sensory activities section), hands at work — fine motor planning (from the fine motor coordination activities section), Let's Doodle activities — pre-writing and pencil control skills (from the pencil to paper section), and the cutting skills section activities were the most important in terms of goal setting. While all activity categories were selected in terms of their worth and importance, the fine motor coordination activities were frequently selected by teachers/teacher aides (28%) as being the most useful in their classrooms.

Of the five teachers/teacher aides who commented on the level of explanation provided for the activities, all indicated they were clearly explained. Seven teachers/teacher aides indicated that suggestions for how to grade activities were helpful. One teacher said, 'Especially useful when I tried activities with [the] whole class — because *everybody* wanted to do Fingergym™!'

Seven teachers/teacher aides responded to questions about their ability to develop their own activities based on activities provided in the manual, the worth and quality of the supplies lists, and the explanation for the set-up of Fingergym™. All indicated that they were pleased with the information provided in the manual. In terms of developing new activities, one teacher/teacher aide responded by saying, 'I have done a few which seemed to work quite well'. When asked whether they felt that they could set up a similar program from the explanations provided in the manual, one teacher responded, 'Using such a great program I could'.

Overwhelmingly, teachers/teacher aides shared with us that both they and the children 'loved' the *Fingergyngles*™ CD, saying things such as, 'Fantastic — we loved it!' and 'Children loved it!'. Of seven teachers/teacher aides participating in the Fingergym™ trials, 86% reported using the three-minute track and 14% reported using the five-minute track. All reported that children were attentive during the silences, and while it was most difficult for preschoolers, they were able to clean up and move on to the next station as the music directed them to.

Although several teachers/teacher aides reported that a four-week trial was not long enough to see clear improvements in fine motor function and behavioural skills, these teachers/teacher aides still felt the program was good and results would be noted in a longer time period. Of those reporting improvement, the most significant were in fine motor coordination and pre-writing and pencil control skills. In the behavioural domain, improvement in self-confidence, independence, and initiative was observed in children participating in the Fingergym™ program.

When asked what teachers/teacher aides liked best about the Fingergym™ program, most responded that the *Fingergyngles*™ CD was the feature they most liked. Other comments included:

'tasks were well categorised'

'children's eagerness to participate'

'book well set out and helpful'

> 'it is a positive program that identifies problems that some children have and sets out how to solve them in a happy and respectful way'
>
> 'The children have enjoyed the program. As a teacher aide the structure was excellent. I always felt I knew exactly what I was doing.'

When asked what they liked least, comments included, '… lots of work changing and organising the materials for activities and it could be expensive', 'the problem of actually setting the activities up in the first place (chasing down resources) then storing these resources', the 'initial set-up always takes a bit of work,' and the pragmatic, 'tidying away the materials'.

A final comment a teacher shared about the Fingergym™ program was, 'Congratulations! The program is sensational. I would like to be able to start the year with this program'.

Glossary

Cognition	'Those processes involving thought and memory; thinking skills'(Westin, 1999, p. G-4).
Fine motor planning	The ability to organise movements and complete activities using the hands and fingers in a smooth and coordinated manner.
Fine motor skills	Those activities requiring coordinated use of the small muscles of the hands.
Graded activity	A task that has the inherent ability to be simplified, and based upon child's ability and motivation can also be made increasingly challenging
Grasp and manipulation skills	Motions that involve use of the hand and fingers in both simple and complex ways.
Gross motor skills	Those skills requiring coordinated use of the large muscles of the body.
In-hand manipulation	'Process of adjusting objects within the hand after grasp' (Exner, 1989, p. 242).
Motor planning (praxis)	Ability to formulate and act upon a plan to carry out a novel motor act (AOTA, 1989).
Muscle strength	'Degree of muscle power when movement is resisted' (AOTA, 1989, p. A-12).
Muscle tone	'Degree of tension or resistance in a muscle' (AOTA, 1989, p. A-12). Muscle tone is often described as low, normal, or high. A child with low muscle tone may appear 'floppy' or loose-limbed, while one with high tone may appear to hold their body in a very rigid manner.
Perception	Interpretation of sensory information in one's environment.
Sensory awareness	Attentiveness to auditory (sound), visual (sight), olfactory (smell), tactile (touch), kinaesthetic (movement), proprioceptive (position of body in space), and vestibular (rotary movement) information.
Sensory defensiveness	An over-reaction to sensory stimuli.
Sensory integration	The organisation of sensory input for use in the environment (Ayres, 1979).
Sensory system parts	Proprioceptive (joint position sense), tactile (touch), kinaesthetic (sense of movement), vestibular (balance), auditory (hearing), visual (sight), olfactory (smell), gustatory (taste)
Visual perception	The ability to interpret and assign meaning to what is seen.
Worker/helper (hands)	An easy way for a child to identify their dominant (worker) hand and non-dominant (helper) hand.

References

American Occupational Therapy Association. (1989). *Guidelines for occupational therapy services in school systems*. Rockville, MD: Author.

Amundson, S. J., & Weil, M. (2001). Prewriting and handwriting skills. In J. Case-Smith (Ed.), *Occupational therapy for children* (4th ed., pp. 545–570). St. Louis, MO: Mosby.

Anderson, T. (2005). Occupational therapy in treating children with developmental delays who have been abused or neglected: A case study. *Australian Occupational Therapy Journal*, *52*(1), 75–77.

Ayres, A. J. (1979). *Sensory integration and the child*. Los Angeles, CA: Western Psychological Services.

Beery, K. (1997). *The Beery-Buktenicz Developmental Test of Visual–Motor Integration* (VMI; 4th ed., Rev.). Parsippany, NJ: Modern Curriculum Press.

Benbow, M. (1995). *Neurokinesthetic approach to hand function and handwriting. Albuquerque,* NM: Clinicians View.

Brigance, A. (1978). *Inventory of early development*. North Billerica, MA: Curriculum Associates.

Case-Smith, J., & Shortridge, S. D. (1996). The developmental process: Prenatal to adolescence. In J. Case-Smith, A. S. Allen & P. N. Pratt (Eds.), *Occupational therapy for children* (3rd ed., pp. 46–66). St. Louis, MO: Mosby.

Cornhill, H., & Case-Smith, J. (1996). Factors that relate to good and poor handwriting. *American Journal of Occupational Therapy, 50*(9), 732–739.

Dankert, H. L., Davies, P. L., & Gavin, W. J. (2003). Occupational therapy effects on visual-motor skills in preschool children. *American Journal of Occupational Therapy, 56*(3), 542–549.

Dennis, J. L., & Swinth, Y. (2001). Pencil grasp and children's handwriting legibility during different-length writing tasks. *American Journal of Occupational Therapy, 55*(2), 175–183.

Edwards, S. J., Buckland, D. B., & McCoy-Powlen, J. D. (2002). *Developmental and functional hand grasps*. Thorofare, NJ: SLACK.

Erhardt, R. P. (1994). *Developmental hand dysfunction: Theory, assessment and treatment* (2nd ed.). Tucson, AZ: Therapy Skill Builders.

Exner, C. (2001). Development of hand skills. In J. Case-Smith (Ed.), *Occupational therapy for children* (4th ed., pp. 289–328). St. Louis, MO: Mosby.

Exner, C. E. (1989). Development of hand functions. In P. N. Pratt & A. S. Allen (Eds.), *Occupational therapy for children* (pp. 235–259). St. Louis, MO: Mosby.

Feder, K., Majnemer, A., & Synnes, A. (2000). Handwriting: Current trends in occupational therapy practice. *Canadian Journal of Occupational Therapy, 67*(3), 197–204.

Furuno, S., O'Reilly, K., Hosaka, C., Inatsuka, T., Zeisloft-Falbey, B., & Allman, T. (1987). *Hawaii early learning profile*. Palo Alto, CA: VORT.

Gesell, A., & Amatruda, C. S. (1947). *Developmental diagnosis* (2nd ed.). New York: Harper and Row.

Hammerschmidt, S. L., & Sudsawad, P. (2004). Teachers' survey on problems with handwriting: Referral, evaluation, and outcomes. *American Journal of Occupational Therapy, 58*(2), 185–192.

Levine, M. (2002). *A mind at a time*. New York: Simon and Schuster.

Losse A., Henderson, S., Elliman, D, Hall, D., Knight, E., & Jongmans, M. (1991). Clumsiness in children: Do they grow out of it? A 10-year follow-up study. *Developmental Medicine and Child Neurology, 33*, 55–68.

Marr, D., Cermak, S., Cohn, E. S., & Henderson, A. (2003). Fine motor activities in Head Start and kindergarten classrooms. *American Journal of Occupational Therapy, 57*(5), 550–557.

Marr, D., & Dimeo, S. B. (2006). Outcomes associated with a summer handwriting course for elementary students. *American Journal of Occupational Therapy, 60*(1), 10–15.

McGarrigle, J. (2006). Evaluating a school skills programme for Australian Indigenous children: A pilot study. *Occupational Therapy International, 13*(1), 1–20.

Shaffer, D. (2002). *Developmental psychology: Childhood and adolescence* (6th ed.). Belmont, CA: Wadsworth.

Skinner, R., & Piek, J. (2001). Psychosocial implications of poor motor control coordination in children and adolescents. *Human Movement Science, 20*, 73–94.

Turner, L., Lammi, B., Friesen, K., & Phelen, N. (2001). *Your child's dressing workbook*. Hamilton, Ontario, Canada: McMaster University, Can*Child* Centre for Child Disability Research.

Westin, D. (1999). *Psychology: Mind, brain and culture*. New York: John Wiley & Sons.

Woodward, S., & Swinth, Y. (2002). Multisensory approach to handwriting remediation: Perceptions of school based occupational therapists. *American Journal of Occupational Therapy, 56*(3), 305–312.

Yakimishyn, J. E., & Magill-Evans, J. (2002). Comparisons among tools, surface orientation and pencil grasp for children 23 months of age. *American Journal of Occupational Therapy, 56*(5), 564–572.

Notes

www.ingramcontent.com/pod-product-compliance
Lightning Source LLC
LaVergne TN
LVHW060213210926
848481LV00008B/2716
* 9 7 8 1 8 7 5 3 7 8 7 5 3 *